Your Health
in America

To cousin Anne,
Be Healthy!
Love, Cousin Wendy

Your Health in America

Problems and Possibilities

Compiled by Wendy Richards

ISBN: 1978172206
ISBN 13: 9781978172203
Library of Congress Control Number: 2017916007
CreateSpace Independent Publishing Platform
North Charleston, South Carolina

BIOGRAPHY

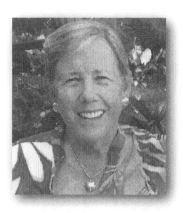

When I was a young teenager, my mother started going to what we all called "witch doctor" classes. Actually they were classes on alternative medicine. Besides learning about vitamins, herbs, and eating right, she learned how to use banana peels to pull out splinters, cayenne pepper paste on paper cuts, cinnamon for a stomach ache, garlic sandwiches for colds, etc. We all laughed at her. But she had the last laugh because she out lived my father by nine years and basically died of a stroke at 93 yrs old with only a medium case of dementia and was otherwise healthy. At least twenty years ago, her doctors were telling her eggs, butter, and high cholesterol were not a problem. But dairy and gluten were.

Over the years, she shared with me the information she learned from her various alternative medicine doctors. I watched her arthritis improve and she never had colds, eyes and ears were fine. She also avoided a knee and hip replacement till she was in her late 80's. She ate no dairy except occasionally goat cheese and had perfect bone density.

As I read and learned more, I changed my diet and steered towards MD's with alternative medicine knowledge. They were more thorough during my office visits and with my blood tests. I was able to get rid of allergies, had fewer colds, my bad gums improved, etc.

Reading, digesting and editing the information in this book into a less technical language has been a labor of love for about 10 years. The more I learned, the more topics I wanted to learn about and share that knowledge with others.

INTRODUCTION

In 2015, The Commonwealth Fund announced that despite the fact that the U. S. spends more on healthcare than any other country in the world, Americans still had poorer health outcomes including shorter life expectancy and greater prevalence of chronic conditions than most of those other countries. Our Western diet is high in animal protein, sugar, and generally processed foods and low on fruits and vegetables and other sources of fiber. Because of these two statements, I decided to call this book Your Health in America not somewhere on another continent.

This book is a compilation of information from many leading natural "alternative medicine" health sources. It is meant to be an introduction to a world of possibilities for your own health. After reading it, I hope you go on to study further by reading some of the books by the authors listed in my sources or checking the internet for more in-depth information. Be careful that any site you visit is up to date and also check that the author is more of an alternative health care thinker.

CHAPTER 1

YOU ARE WHAT YOU EAT!

Tell me what you eat, and I will tell you who you are.
A. BRILLAT SAVARIN (1755-1826)

The food industry, with its billions of advertising and marketing dollars, tries to convince us to eat its dairy, meat, fish, poultry, and eggs as well as their products often laden with sugar, salt, and fats. This constant assault convinces the public to eat foods that can make them either fat and/or sick. Obesity, high blood pressure, diabetes, heart disease, cancer, arthritis, multiple sclerosis, lupus, gallstones, diverticulitis, osteoporosis, allergies, and asthma are but a sampling of the diseases resulting from the "Western diet". The link between diet and health is not well understood by the public or most medical doctors. Nutrition is very important in preventing and recovering from disease! Most physicians don't know anything about nutrition. Many patients are nutritionally deficient when they are admitted to the hospital. In the hospital it gets worse, especially in intensive care. Pneumonia and urinary infections are a common result. Many doctors were not even required to take a nutrition course in medical school. Fortunately this is gradually changing. What most traditional doctors don't know is that "alternative medicine" is based on hard science from some of the best researchers and laboratories in the world. Also, the pharmaceutical industry, which promotes the use of drugs over food for maintaining health, has a powerful lobby in Washington, D.C. Simply put, these industries control our nutritional thinking and there is little or no money in it for them when we eat right and consequently remain healthy.

One of the best things you can personally do for your own health is to put the most wholesome food in your body. "Whole" is the operative word in that sentence. Eating food that is as close to the way Mother Nature made it - like: fresh fruits, vegetables, whole grains, legumes (beans, lentils, peas), some meats or fish, plain yogurt, cheese, eggs, olive oil or coconut oil, herbs and spices. Think basically a Mediterranean diet. Avoid foods that are refined, processed, artificial, and/or have chemical additives in them. Eating good carbs which are whole grains like brown, red or black rice, quinoa, farro, kamut, millet, oats, and barley in moderation will NOT make you gain weight (and will also give you a good helping of fiber as well as the vitamins and minerals in them). If you eat a varied diet, you don't have to worry about missing one or another vitamin or mineral. In general it is better to get your vitamins and minerals from your food itself (as opposed to supplements). Also, using non-iodized sea salt will give you 48 minerals while not affecting your blood pressure.

Protein:

Protein is important in our diet. The amino acids in protein are needed by our bodies for growth, repair of muscles, formation of essential digestive enzymes, immune system function, and to make hormones. It helps to build lean body mass (your weight minus the fat) that gives you an efficient engine to burn calories that in turn raises your basal metabolic rate (the rate at which your body burns calories while at rest while still keeping your vital functions going such as breathing and maintaining warmth). We all need protein but we don't need as much protein as we have been led to believe. Our bodies need less than 2 oz of protein a day. That protein can come from meat, fish, dairy, or vegetables and legumes.

Sitting down to a 6 oz piece of meat for dinner is the equivalent of 3 days of your protein needs and contains fat, cholesterol, and (if not organically raised) carcinogens, hormones, antibiotics, etc. Most of our beef, chicken, pork, turkey, etc. is raised in factory-style farms where the suppliers raise the largest number of animals, with the idea of maximum efficiency and speed, to maturity/slaughter. They are fed artificial growth hormones to help them grow faster and, in the case of dairy cows, produce more milk. The animals are also fed antibiotics and packed as tightly as possible in their pens or cages. I won't go into what happens at the slaughterhouse. The United States, which has 5 percent of the world's population, raises and kills about 20 percent of the animals consumed worldwide for food. The methane gas created by these cows creates more greenhouse gases than all the CO_2 derived from cars and trucks. Large forested areas around the world are being cleared to raise cattle. Waste from animals is not treated in sanitation plants but spread onto the land and then much of it runs off and pollutes the nearby streams and groundwater. A great deal of land and water are also needed to raise the grains to feed these animals. These grains are filled with herbicides and pesticides to help them grow more quickly. About 50% of the fresh water in the United States is used, one way or another, for raising animals for food. Soil erosion is another concern with more than half of the topsoil in the western states having already been lost. If you still feel you want to eat meat, fish and dairy products, then consume only the organic versions grown on smaller farms because they are fed non GMO grains, and organic feeds, and have no antibiotics or hormones in them. Grass fed beef with no hormones is the best - but eating any beef still contributes to many of the problems mentioned above.

Fish are not much better, with the most common ones (tuna & swordfish) having mercury and/or PCB's in them. Farmed salmon is fed pellets of chicken feces, corn meal, soy, and chemicals to make them pink, and other pulverized fish containing concentrations of toxins. Farmed salmon has 7 times the levels of PCB's as wild salmon and less omega 3's due to their lack of a wild diet. Crowding inhibits their movement and causes disease so they are also fed high levels of antibiotics. According to the Monterey Bay Aquarium seafood watch guides, the best fish to eat are: Alaskan <u>wild</u> salmon, albacore tuna (if it is pole or troll caught from the U.S. or British Columbia and has the Marine Stewardship Council blue eco label on the can), farmed oysters, Pacific wild sardines, farmed rainbow trout (which is not sitting in a polluted stream but a freshwater pond and they are fed a better diet of fishmeal), freshwater farmed Coho salmon (these are raised in freshwater pens and require less feed so the environmental impacts are reduced. All these "good" meats, fish, eggs, and dairy products also contain an amino acid called leucine which also helps regulate another beneficial "anti aging" enzyme known as TOR.

We don't have to eat meat, fish, or dairy products to get all the essential amino acids we need. They are also found in soy products, grains, legumes, vegetables, and some fruits as well. We need to eat "complete proteins". Protein is formed by amino acid building blocks. There are 20 different amino acids that form a protein molecule and 9 of those are called "essential" because they cannot be made by our body- we need to eat them. Meat, fish, and dairy are "complete" proteins but beans and nuts are not - but we don't need essential amino acids in every bite of food in every meal. We only need a sufficient amount of each amino acid every day. The best complete proteins are: quinoa, buckwheat, soy, rice & beans, Ezekiel bread, pita & hummus, peanut butter & bread or cracker, spirulina, chia seeds, nuts. Plant based diets contain a wide variety of amino acids. No matter what kind of diet we eat, we must always eat a "varied diet" to get enough protein, vitamins, and minerals.

Grain Brain book Good Pantry items

Fats:

coconut oil
olive oil
sesame oil
Irish butter
ghee
almond milk

avocado
olives
nuts and butters
cheese (no blue)
seeds

Herbs and Seasonings:

mustard
tapenades
salsa
herbs
seasonings

Low Sugar Fruits:

avocado
bell pepper
cucumber
tomatoes, zucchini
squash
pumpkin
eggplant
lemons
limes

Protein:

eggs
wild fish

shellfish
grass fed meat
poultry
all meats

Legumes:

hummus

Vegetables:

all green and leafy
onions
mushrooms
radishes
turnips
garlic
ginger
jicama
water chestnuts

In Moderation:

carrots
parsnips
cottage cheese
yogurt
milk and cream
beans, lentils, peas

Non Gluten Grains:

buckwheat
rice
quinoa
oats (but check that it's gluten free)
stevia
dark chocolate at least 70%
berries
red wine (1 glass)

Water:
Our bodies are 75% water so drink it - **but not with meals** - as it dilutes your digestive juices. Have a big glass first thing in the morning because you are dehydrated from sleeping all night. Drink a glass 30 minutes before lunch and dinner and one just before bed. Space your drinking throughout the day. Coffee, salty meats, soy sauce, popcorn, fried foods, sugary drinks (like Coke or Pepsi) and alcohol are dehydrating. If exercising, remember to drink water also to rehydrate.

Salt:
Sodium is a vital nutrient in your body because it maintains the levels of fluids and provides channels for nerve signaling. We cannot live without it. Commercial salt is not complete salt. It is refined and some of the natural minerals are removed. Unrefined salt has more than 80 minerals including magnesium & potassium that help with normal blood pressure. Refined table salt has been dyed white with bleach and anti clumping agents that have been added, as well as aluminum, to help with shelf life. Too much salt can raise your blood pressure. Eating processed foods, fast foods, and canned foods gives us too much salt. On the other hand, a low sodium diet

is not good either. Low sodium diets can harm your blood vessels, cause deficiencies of calcium and deplete vitamin B vitamins. When eating salt, stick to the natural sea salt with their natural minerals and not "table salt" having all those bad additives.

Iodine:

Iodine is necessary for good thyroid function and a good metabolism. Foods rich in iodine are: seaweed, fish, shellfish, shrimp, cod, sea bass, and haddock. Iodized salt is not as good as it sounds because there is little iodine in it and that iodine is not bio-available. Symptoms of low iodine are: brittle nails, cold hands and feet, dry skin, hair loss, fatigue, weight gain, etc.

Calcium:

Among the public, getting enough calcium is a big concern these days. The dairy lobby has convinced us that "milk does a body good" but that couldn't be further from the truth. After babies have been weaned from their mother's milk, mammals (that's us too) have no need for any kind of milk or the casein in it. Casein is the primary protein in dairy products, which has also been identified as one of the most potent chemical carcinogens. The highest incidents of breast cancer and osteoporosis are in those countries with the highest dairy product consumption - Finland, Sweden, USA, and England. Eating animal protein, table salt and drinking coffee contributes to calcium loss through your urine. When was the last time you ate any dairy products in a Chinese, Japanese, Thai, Vietnamese, or Indian restaurant? These cultures don't eat dairy and consequently have lower rates of osteoporosis and other bone diseases. They also eat meat and fish more sparingly, as condiments. Here is a list, in descending order, of the foods having the best rate of calcium absorption in your body: Brussels sprouts, mustard greens, broccoli, turnip greens, kale, and finally cow's milk! One cup of milk does contain 300mg of calcium but only 96mg of it is bio-available to us. Eat 1.5 cups of cooked broccoli and you get the same amount of bio-available calcium. Cow's milk comes obviously from cows (ie: meat protein) - do you see a vicious cycle here? The more milk you drink, the more calcium you loose through urination. If you feel like you need a calcium supplement, there is one on the market made by the Pioneer Co. that is plant based. Almond or cashew milk contain more calcium in them that is bioavailable without added sugar. I'm told Silk is the better product than Blue Diamond and is also available in a no sugar added version. Picture an African savannah with a herd of cape buffalos, giraffes, and rhinoceroses that are the strongest boned animals on earth. Where are they getting their calcium? They get it from the grass they eat.

Soy:
People who are not eating meat often turned to soy as an alternate protein source. Soy protein, especially unfermented soy protein (tofu, soy milk, soy beans) contains the highest amount of phytic acid of any known substance. This acid blocks mineral absorption: especially zinc, but also calcium, copper, zinc, magnesium, and iron. Only a long period of fermentation will significantly reduce the phytate content of soybeans. The soybean contains a clot promoting substance, which makes red blood cells stick together or "clump". Fermentation can deactivate this substance. Only one ounce of soy protein consumed daily can cause breast abnormalities due to soy's powerfully estrogenic effects. Soy formula for babies contains 100 times more aluminum than unprocessed milk. Aluminum is toxic to the nervous system and kidneys. Babies exclusively fed soy formula receive the estrogen equivalent of at least five birth control pills per day. Many girls show signs of puberty before the age of 8. Soy foods increase the body's requirement for vitamin D. The Asians consume mainly fermented soy products as condiments such as tempeh, natto, tamari, and soy sauce.

Fats:

We all need fat in our diet because it lubricates the bone joints, it helps reduce inflammation, regulates the immune system, 70% of the brain is made up of fat, helps with brain function too. Fat is needed to help fat soluble vitamins get absorbed. The only fats that you should eat are extra virgin olive oil, organic or raw butter, ghee, avocado, and coconut oil. Do not cook with olive oil or butter as heating them changes them into a trans fat in your body. Antioxidants are needed then to make them chemically not carcinogenic. Coconut oil had been used as cooking oil for thousand of years. There is even coconut oil mayonnaise now called Coconaise. Then came the anti-saturated fat campaign and the promotion of polyunsaturated fats such as canola, soybean, safflower, corn, and margarine. Saturated fats were supposedly linked to high cholesterol and heart disease. Most Americans eat a diet high in unsaturated fats and yet have a very high rate of both diseases. Excess amounts of polyunsaturated fats in our diet are central to the development of many degenerative diseases. To name a few: cancer, heart disease, arthritis, immunodeficiency, diabetes, hypertension, osteoporosis, and connective tissue disease. The harmful effects of unsaturated oil lie in their unsaturation, which causes the oil to become rancid inside the body. Commercial meats have unsaturated fats because the animals are fed soybeans and corn, both high in unsaturated fats.

Omega 3 fat is another nutrient that is important to our general health. In the past, our meat, dairy products, and eggs were a good source of this nutrient. Not so now except for free range chicken eggs. Not all "free range" eggs are created equal though (but the non profit organization called Cornucopia Institute's web site: www.cornucopia.org has a great chart that rates all of the organic egg producers in the country). Your best bet is trying to buy your eggs at the local farmer's market or health food store. Eggs have gotten a bad rap in relation to heart disease and cholesterol. Every cell in your body needs cholesterol. It helps to make hormones, vitamin D, strengthen cell membrane, bile acids that help you digest your food, and neurological function. There are numerous studies that have concluded that eggs have nothing to do with raising your cholesterol anyway. Eggs are the best source of high quality protein (the whites). The yolks contain phospholipids that are beneficial for all cells and lutein. Lutein protects eyes against macular degeneration and protects the retina from blue light waves that are damaging to the eye also. Omega-3 oils are also plentiful in flax seeds, flax seed oil, chia seeds and in fatty fish (salmon, herring, mackerel, and sardines) and in lesser amounts in walnuts, hemp seeds, green leafy vegetables and canola oil. Flax seed oil has an advantage over fish oil as fatty fish are full of mercury and other environmental contaminates. Flax seed oil also has a particular type of Omega-3 called ALA that the body needs and plant fiber that has been associated with reduced incidences of breast, colon, and prostate cancer.

Organic foods:
Organic foods contain from 200-400% more minerals than commercial foods. Produce can be called organic if it has grown in soil that has had no prohibited substances (synthetic fertilizers and pesticides) applied to it in the past 3 years.

Why cooked foods are better for you:
Nutrients in raw foods are difficult to release with the normal amount of chewing. A class of compounds that are called flavonoids are import for slowing and reversing the age related degeneration of the brain. These compounds are released when foods are cooked. High flavonoid foods are: broccoli, celery, chocolate, citrus fruits, ginkgo biloba, leeks, onions, parsley, berries, red wine, tea, tomatoes, turmeric, and walnuts. Steaming vegetables is the best way to cook them. Some vegetables contain compounds that can cause joint pain (peppers) and suppresses thyroid function (kale, broccoli, Brussels sprouts) when eaten raw. Cooking them destroys the harmful compounds.

Super Foods:

These are foods that are superior sources of antioxidants that help protect the body's cells from the harmful effects of free radicals. Free radical damage is linked to cancer, heart disease, Alzheimer's and Parkinson's as well as the aging process. They are: chia seeds, acai berries, goji berries, maca, and hemp.

Chia seeds:

These tiny black seeds come from a plant in the mint family and have massive amounts of nutrients packed in a low calorie and low carbohydrate package. You will find quality protein, antioxidants, omega 3 fatty acids, and fiber. Eating these can help with type II diabetes, improve bone health, improve exercise workout results. They are easy to add to many foods and when wet, swell up and soften so they can be used as thickeners in recipes.

Acai berries:

These berries come from the Amazon rainforest. They taste like a cross between a blueberry and a grape and are best if they have been freeze dried quickly after picking and then made into drinks, etc. They are chock full of antioxidants.

Gogi berries (wolf berries):

These berries are widely grown throughout Asia and taste like a cross between a cranberry and a cherry. They are a rich source of vitamin A, B1, B2, B6, C, and E and contain a full compliment of protein.

Maca:

A turnip like root grown in Peru that is made into a powder and was eaten by the Incas for 2,000 years to increase their strength, endurance, and libido.

Hemp:

Hemp is related to the mulberry and has a rich nutty flavor. It is a complete protein and has more than 20 trace minerals and the oil is almost as powerful as vitamin E and it contains a lot of zinc. This is the seed of the hemp "marijuana" plant but these seeds do not have enough THC to give you a "high".

Cruciferous vegetables:

These vegetables have very powerful health promoting elements. They include: Brussels sprouts, cauliflower, broccoli, cabbage, and kale. They contain high concentrations of beneficial nutrients that have been studied extensively because of their ability to inhibit cancer growth. In addition, researchers have discovered broccoli protects the heart and brain. Make sure to steam it and not eat it raw to release these benefits.

Teas:

Teas contain a number of beneficial compounds particularly catechin which may reduce stroke, heart failure, cancer, and diabetes. Green tea contains about 30% catechin and amounts are even higher in white tea. Black tea is not as exciting. Tea is also a good source of quercetin a potent anti-inflammatory flavonoid that also fights cancer and protects the brain. Unfortunately, tea also contains high levels of two toxins: fluoride and aluminum. The good news is that little of the aluminum is absorbed by the body because it it bound by catechin. The bad news is adding citrus like lemon juice to it dramatically increases aluminum absorption by 700%. Try flavoring your tea with mint instead. White tea has more catechin and far less fluoride and aluminum.

Vitamins:

Vitamins come in two varieties: water soluble and fat soluble. Water soluble vitamins, such as B complex vitamins and vitamin C dissolve in water and are excreted through the kidneys (if there is an excess in your body). Fat soluble vitamins like A, D, E and K dissolve in the fat and are stored in fat throughout the body. It is difficult for your body to excrete excess fat soluble vitamins, so toxic levels can accumulate if you consume too many. Before taking any supplements, it is smart to get the advice of your physician or professional pharmacist as it is tricky to get synergy.

Vitamin A:

Plays a part in bone growth, reproduction and the immune system health. It also helps the skin and mucous membranes repel bacteria and viruses more effectively and is essential to healthy vision. Some of the best sources of vitamin A include eggs, milk, carrots, yellow and orange vegetables, spinach and other leafy green vegetables. It is a fat soluble vitamin so you can overdose on it.

B Vitamins:

There are 8 B vitamins and they are all water soluble and they play an important role in cell metabolism. They are chemically distinct but are referred to in dietary supplements as vitamin B complex. Vitamin B-12 is a crucial vitamin necessary for the proper functioning of the brain and the nervous system. Most people get this vitamin from eating meat or other animal based foods. B-12 actually comes from a type of bacteria that is in the soil and water in which the plants grow that the animals then eat. Plant eating animals have always gotten this vitamin from the dirt that clung to the nooks and crannies on their fruits and vegetables. Today, our food is so sanitized that we never get this dirt. The safe thing to do if you want to be a vegetarian is to take a natural B-12 supplement.

Choline:

Choline or vitamin B 4 is good for the brain and is in eggs, dairy, toasted wheat germ, peanut butter, almonds, oat bran, codfish, beef, turkey, and chicken.

Vitamin C:

This vitamin was historically important in the treatment of scurvy. These days, it is used for the treatment of colds and to boost the immune system, lowering hypertension. It is an anti-inflammatory so it is good to take right after exercise to help with pain. Signs of vitamin C deficiency include dry hair, gingivitis and bleeding gums, easy bruising, difficulty with wound healing. Some of the best sources of the vitamin are: peppers, dark green leafy greens, kiwi, broccoli, berries, citrus, tomatoes, peas, papaya, guava.

Vitamin D:

We get our vitamin D from the sun and it is added to some of our foods. Seniors especially need this vitamin (actually a brain hormone) because it lowers the risk of osteoporosis and other bone disorders. It helps them keep their mobility and independence. It can decrease the risk of cardiovascular problems, diabetes and some cancers and helps with calcium absorption (which is why it is often added to dairy products). Vitamin D also helps our immune system by boosting our T cells that are a type of white blood cells. White blood cells help you fight colds and flu.

Vitamin E:

It is a fat soluble antioxidant which can protect against toxins such as air pollution and eye disorders such as cataracts. It is necessary for structural and functional maintenance of the skeletal, cardiac, and muscle parts of the body. It also assists in the formation of red blood cells and helps to maintain stores of vitamins A, K, minerals iron and selenium. It has a positive effect on the immune system, protects against heart disease, cancer, relieves symptoms of Alzheimer's disease and may help prevent some diabetes related damage, especially to the eyes. It also helps shore up nerves and prevents peripheral neuropathy. Food sources are vegetable oils, avocados, spinach, sunflower seeds, wheat germ, nuts, and whole grains.

Vitamin K: see heart attack paragraph in Chapter# 2

Magnesium:

It plays an important role in our bodies. It helps with calcium absorption, blood pressure regulation, reduces inflammation, raises brain cell antioxidant glutathione levels, helps with protein synthesis, nerve function, blood sugar control, neurotransmitter release, energy metabolism. Magnesium rich foods are: leafy green vegetables, pumpkin seeds, yogurt, almonds, black beans, avocado figs, dark chocolate, bananas, salmon, cashews, coriander, goat cheese, and artichokes. Magnesium can help with: cardiovascular disease, fibromyalgia, type 2 diabetes, osteoporosis, and migraine headaches. For best absorption, take with B complex vitamins, vitamin D, and selenium. Magnesium protects the brain after a stroke by helping blood flow and reducing inflammation.

Zinc:

Taking zinc supports your immune system. Many types of cold remedies contain zinc. If you feel a cold coming on, you can take a simple zinc supplement several times a day for a few days and it will stop your cold from getting worse.

Omega 3 & 6 & 9:

Another nutrient that is important for general health is Omega-3 fats. Our bodies convert the Omega-3 into DHA that is a nutrient that is needed by all of us but is especially critical for the development of the brain in fetuses and in newborns. (see the fats section above) Both omega 3 & 6 cannot be made by our bodies so must be taken through supplements of our food. Omega 9 can be synthesized in our body and is in olive, canola, peanut, and safflower oils.

Iodine:

Iodine is necessary for good thyroid function and metabolism function. Foods that are rich in iodine are: seaweed, shrimp, fish (haddock, cod, sea bass), and shellfish. Iodized salt does not have much iodine in it and this form is not bioavailable. Sea salt has no iodine but has a lot of minerals in it. Some symptoms of low iodine are brittle nails, cold hands & feet, dry skin, hair loss, fatigue, goiter, weight gain, etc. Low iodine can kill your thyroid.

"Off the radar/wall" supplements:

Moringa arborea:

Moringa is considered a super food in Asia. It is made from several parts of a flowering plant in the Moringacae family endemic to Kenya but grown in many tropical countries and has antioxidants, anti-inflammatories, amino acids, vitamins and minerals. It has 7 times more vitamin C than oranges, 4 times the calcium in milk, 4 times the vitamin A in carrots, 3 times the potassium in bananas, 2 times the protein in yogurt, more chlorophyll than dark leafy green vegetables, and anti cancer properties.

Bacopa:

Bacopa is a natural herbal plant containing an antioxidant compound that can improve memory, reduce inflammation, is an antidepressant, and even helps with Parkinson's disease, Alzheimer's and stroke. Note that it can take up to 6 weeks or so to build up in your system to have an effect.

Taurine:

Taurine is an amino acid that is the most abundant amino acid in the body but especially high in the brain, retina, and heart. The heart has both taurine and another amino acid called glutamate. Too much glutamate can make the heart irritable, leading to arrhythmia. Taurine counteracts heart muscle excitation to prevent this from happening. The chance of ventricular fibrillation that is a major cause of death following a heart attack is reduced drastically if the patient is given taurine. It can help improve the effectiveness of traditional arrhythmia medicine. In the brain, it plays a major role in stimulating stem cells that are important for brain repair even in older adults. One of the most important ways taurine helps the brain is by reducing inflammation. If you already have heart disease, taking daily supplements to keep your level of this important amino acid high. Another added bonus is how taurine can help with hearing loss. Damage to the cochlea in the ear happens with age and recent studies have found that taurine can stimulate cochlear stem cells and improve their ability to survive which means your hearing could improve. It comes in capsule form but is water soluble so the powder from the capsule can be mixed with water and taken that way which may be easier than taking a lot of capsules. Taking taurine during chemo therapy treatment can also help diminish some side effects.

Things that are not so good for you:

MSG (Mono sodium glutamate):

Monosodium Glutamate is the sodium salt of glutamic acid and is one of the most abundant naturally occurring non-essential amino acids. It is found in tomatoes, Parmesan cheese, potatoes, mushrooms and other vegetables and fruits. In the food manufacturing plant process the bound glutamate is broken down and made into a "free protein" by various processes. When this different glutamate, now know as D-glutamate, is isolated and eaten separately, it spikes glutamate acid which causes brain damage in babies. MSG used to be in baby food. Some people are more sensitive to MSG than others. It can cause obesity, has been associated with neurodegenerative diseases, neurodevelopmental abnormalities, nervous system injury, endocrine disorders, diabetes I & II, cancer growth and spread, sudden cardiac death, GI disorders, lupus and other auto immune disorders, atherosclerosis, retinal disorders, and immune dysfunction. Most of the effects of MSG occur silently and accumulate over a number of years. Studies have shown that when you combine foods containing MSG with those containing aspartame, blood glutamate levels are twice as high as they would be if you ate the MSG alone! Think chips or a frozen dinner and diet soda. People do this all the time. Check food labels as there are many common disguised names for MSG and portobello mushrooms are naturally high in glutamic acid - the harmful component of MSG.

Sulfites:
Sulfites are a kind of food additive that are used in the food processing industry to preserve foods. They protect foods from such things as spoilage, loss of flavor, and bacterial growth in wines. Migraine headaches can most commonly be caused by sulfites in wine, cheese and chocolate. High sulfite levels in the blood and tissues inhibit an enzyme that keeps brain glutamate levels down. Avoid wine that contains sulfites, especially white wine. Foods that contain higher levels of sulfites are: beer, dried fruits, guacamole, molasses, shrimp, soup mixes, jams, cider, beet sugar, corn sweeteners, gelatin. Vitamin E can block the toxic effects of sulfites but not the impairment of learning and memory.

Gluten:
When you eat gluten, the digestion process by your body makes a compound like morphine so you feel like you are on some kind of opiate! no wonder why so many people have troubles staying off bread, pasta and pastries, etc. Humans never ate gluten until about 10,000 years ago (and that is relatively recently in our human race's history!). The grains early humans ate were different from what we eat today because of seed hybridization

and genetic modification. The body negatively reacts to gluten by interfering with the breakdown and absorption of nutrients. The body sends out an inflammatory message "there is an enemy in here"! Gluten sensitivity is found commonly in people with neurological diseases because of the inflammation connection. But, they can have these diseases without any gastrointestinal problems. Diabetes, Alzheimer's, depression, arthritis, insomnia, intestinal problems, mood disorders, and obesity to name a few are caused by inflammation! 40% of the population cannot process gluten and the rest are in harm's way.

gluten grains:

barley
bulgar
coucous
farina
graham flour
matzo
rye
semolina
spelt
triticale
wheat
wheat germ

foods with gluten:

baked beans (canned)
beer
bouillon/broths
cereals

chocolate milk (store)
cold cuts
egg substitute
energy bars
flavored coffee/tea
French fries
fruit fillings/puddings
gravy
hot dogs
ice cream
imitation bacon/crabmeat
instant hot drinks
ketchup
malt
marinades
mayonnaise
meatballs /meatloaf (store)
non- dairy creamer
oat bran (unless certified free)
oats (unless certified free)
processed cheeses like Velveeta

gluten free grains:

amaranth
arrowroot
buckwheat
corn
millet
potato
quinoa
rice

sorghum
soy
tapioca
roasted nuts
root beer
salad dressings
sausage
seitan
soups
soy sauce/ teriyaki sauce
syrups
tabbouleh
trail mix
veggie burgers
vodka
wheatgrass
wine coolers

misc. sources of gluten

cosmetics
lipstick/ lip balm
medications
shampoos/ conditioners
vitamins/ supplements (check label)

alternative words for gluten:

amino peptide complex
avena sativa
brown rice syrup

caramel coloring
cyclodextrin
fermented grain extract
hordeum distichon
hordeum vulgare
hydrolysate
hydrolyzed malt extract
hydrolized vegetable protein
maltodextrin
modified food starch
natural flavoring
phytosphingosine extract
secale cereale
soy protein
triticum aestivum
triticum vulgare
vegetable protein (HVP)
yeast extract

Artificial sweeteners:

Aspartame or NutraSweet was added to diet soda in the 1980's by some soda companies to replace Sweet & Lo in their carbonated beverages because it was causing bad side effects in many people. At the same time, researchers said there was a problem with NutraSweet having bad side effects too, but the FDA ignored them - as well as the complaints from the general public. Some people experienced headaches, memory loss, vision problems, dizziness, insomnia, diarrhea, nightmares, and nausea to name a few. Diet soda with aspartame is especially bad for children whose brains are still forming. It can be addictive. Dr. Russell Blaylock says it can bring on stronger symptoms of MS, Parkinson's, Alzheimer's and other neuromuscular diseases. Formaldehyde is one of the toxins that stay in your body when Aspartame breaks down. When Stevia, a natural sweetener from South America, was made available in the USA, the FDA fought its use as a sweetener! Aspartame is still being used in many foods. Another safer sugar substitute is called Just Like Sugar. It is made from a natural dietary fiber derived from chicory root, flavors extracted from orange peel, etc. Give it a try. To protect yourself against the free radicals that are caused by excitotoxins from this chemical in your brain, take antioxidants as well as vitamins E, D, and C, magnesium citrate, antioxidant enzymes, zinc, selenium, melatonin.

Sucralose, one of the ingredients in Splenda, was discovered in England by a company named Tate & Lyle. A scientist was working on a substitute for DDT. He thought if he could add chlorine to sucrose the new chemical formed with these partially chlorinated sugars would contain carbon-chlorine bonds like DDT. But unlike DDT, the partially chlorinated sugars dissolved in water and suffered bio-degradation. The "party line" from their partner McNeil Nutritionals, LLC that now makes it in USA, is that none of the Splenda stays in your body. Actually, even the FDA admits that 11 to 27% stays in your body. Other adverse effects are: gastrointestinal problems, seizures, dizziness, migraines, allergic reactions, blood sugar increases and weight gain. It can interfere with the efficacy of drugs you are taking. It is not safe for cooking either as it's touted. Another ingredient in Splenda is Dextrose that is made from corn (see GMO's section) and is used when necessary in hospitals to increase a person's blood sugar. Just use real sugar if you need to sweeten your food. Some people who live in southern states, where there are sugar ants, use Splenda sprinkled near their paths to kill them. It works!

GMO foods:
John Robbins stated the purpose of growing GM foods was to increase crop yields, reduce costs for farmers and to use less amounts of herbicides. None of these things happened. People around the world have joined forces to

refuse GM foods because of the dangers they represent to human health. Europe eliminated them from their food supply about 10 years ago.

GMO foods can contribute to food allergies, cause damage to your immune system, and cause cancer. An estimated 75% of the food in our grocery stores contains GM ingredients. It doesn't help to look at the labels because no labeling for GM products is required in most states. Most soy and feed corn grown in the USA is GMO and as a result, so are the processed foods made from them. Some side products that you wouldn't think were from GMO foods are: maltodextrin, soy lecithin, and high fructose corn syrup, rennet used to make hard cheese, aspartame, and milk containing rBGH (bovine growth hormone used to increase milk production)

Stay away from them. Monsanto who makes many of them rigged their testing to make them appear safe for us to eat. There is actually a chemical "dumbing down" of America going on right now because so many of the chemicals in our food are toxic to our brains. The general public believes what the government tells them when it comes to many things but many feel the government has lied to them in the past and continue to do so now. Do not believe what the FDA says because they are being paid by big Pharma companies and other food producing companies who have lobbyists all over Washington D.C. Many members of the FDA governing boards also sit on Big Pharma boards of directors.

The True Food Shopping Guide (see sources) is a great tool to help you learn which brands and products contain GMO ingredients.

Microwave ovens:

Originally, microwave ovens were developed by the Nazis to use as part of mobile support operations during WW II. After the war, the Soviet Union retrieved some of these microwave ovens and did the most thorough research on their biological effects. As a result, their use was purportedly outlawed around 1976 - but then subsequently lifted. Dr. Lita Lee, PhD says microwave ovens affect the food as well as the people who eat the food. Microwaving causes adverse affects in food such as the formation of cancer-causing sub-stances, leakage of toxic chemicals from the packaging into the food and de-struction of nutrients. What happens to people who ingest microwave foods or who are exposed to external sources of microwave radiation? Carcinogens were found in virtually all food tested by Russian investigators. They also found the nutritive value of the microwave foods to decrease by 60% to 90%. The packaging used for the foods leaked carcinogenic chemicals into the food. Health effects noticed by the researchers included: lymphatic dis-orders, increased rate of cancer cell formation, increased rate of stomach and intestinal cancers, and a high rate of digestive disorders.

Acid – Alkaline balance:

Our bodies are alkaline by design and acid by function. The greatest weap-on for fighting bacteria growth and disease such as cancer in our bodies is an alkaline body. The pH balance of our body is the first line of defense for your immune system. Cellular activity creates acid and this acid gives cells energy and function. The body works hard not to let these acids build up and maintain a balanced pH. We upset this balance by eating acid foods like meat, sugar, dairy products, as well as the highly acid chemicals like preservatives, additives, artificial sweeteners, chloride and fluoride in tap water. Fat is used in our bodies to buffer the effect of acids. We hold on to the fat and store it until it can be eliminated in our urine. Various minerals are also necessary to buffer the acids and if we don't have enough of them, calcium is pulled from the bones (causing osteoporosis) and magnesium from the muscles. Another buffering system is the lymphatic one. This lymphatic fluid is pumped by the movements of our muscles. A sedentary lifestyle leads to the build up of acid in the tissues. When you look at an acid/alkaline chart on the Internet, you may see foods you think are acid or alkaline on the wrong side of it. The foods are placed on the chart by how they affect urine pH. A balanced diet contains 20% acid forming foods and 80% alkaline. In the same turn, if you are taking calcium or magnesium (that are common in antacids, as they neutralize the stomach acids) this makes your body too alkaline. Hard water is full of minerals and tends to be alkaline. Soft water tends to be more acid. The main thing to remember is to try to keep a balanced pH in your body.

Alkaline forming foods:

> 80% of your daily diet should contain these foods:
> All vegetables except dried beans, lentils, asparagus tips, and garbanzos
> All fresh fruits except cranberries, plums, prunes, blueberries (preserves and canned fruits are actually acid forming)
> Almonds, chestnuts, Brazil nuts, and hazelnuts

Acid forming foods:

> 20% of your daily diet should contain these foods:
> All meats except beef juice and bone meal
> All grains, cereals and bakery goods except for soybeans
> All dairy products except buttermilk, yogurt, raw milk and whey
> Peanuts, pecans, and walnuts

Certain food combinations are difficult to digest and may cause problems in the digestive system.

Here is a brief list of food combinations to avoid:

> Two or more starchy foods at the same meal
> Sugary foods and starchy foods
> Milk and citrus
> Cereals and citrus
> Large quantities of starchy food with meat or cheese
> Coffee with milk or cream
> Raw apples with other foods

Why We Get Fat by Gary Taubes

The American accepted thinking about weight gain and loss changed in the 70's when fat was accused of causing heart problems. These scientists decided weight gain was an eating disorder, a psychological problem. What we have been taught to think in the last 40 years: calories in / calories out. The more we eat and the less exercise we do, the fatter we get. Actually, the way it really works is: if our food/fuel is restricted, our energy is less - we slow down and we burn fewer calories and this limits weight loss. We get hungrier so that when more food is again available, we eat more and gain back the few pounds we lost and more. Think the "yo-yo" effect we have all seen. Gluttony and sloth is in our heads - lack of will power, laziness, etc. causes our failure to stay thin.

The cavemen ate mostly meat and fat and some wild vegetables, nuts and fruits (berries) that had carbs but they were high fiber carbs. Our bodies were designed to store fat because we didn't know when the next meal would be "coming around the corner". 60% of our modern diet was not invented or around until recently in history. Peoples around the world, whether meat eaters or vegetarians, don't get obese or "Western" diseases because none of them eat white flour, cereal grains, dairy products, sweetened beverages, vegetable oil and dressings, sugar, or candy. Eating less total fat and saturated fat and replacing these with vegetables, fruits and whole grains have shown to have no beneficial effects at all as far as heart disease, stroke, breast cancer, colon cancer, etc or weight gain.

If calories don't count, then what does cause us to gain weight? Eating too many carbohydrates, our hormones, certain enzymes and our genetics. Carbohydrates: flours, pasta, cereal grains, starchy vegetables, all sugars, beer, fruit, fruit juice, and sodas. Most foods except, meat, fish, dairy, and fats have some amount of carbs.

Hormones and enzymes play a big part that will be explained below. Genetics also plays a big role. Genetics determine our body height and weight. (Think animals that are bred for being fatter or larger.) We eat to get to that predetermined size. As children we don't get tall or fat because we overeat, we overeat because we are growing.

Animals don't need excessive amounts of food to make needed fat. They do it for a reason like for hibernating, for long migrations (birds, whales), on a schedule-seasonally like bears and squirrels. This weight gain is genetic/evolutionary. Regulating of fat is done normally. If something happens to throw off the natural regulation of fat in their tissues, health problems arise.

Now for some biology: Fat is continually flowing in and out of our fat cells and circulating around to be used for fuel. If it is not used, it is returned to the cells for later use. Our cells burn carbs before they burn fat because they are a quicker source of energy and blood sugar regulation. If there are no carbs around to burn, the body will burn fat! The hormone, insulin, keeps our blood sugar under control. We actually loose fat while sleeping because we are not eating food/fuel to replace it. The hormones estrogen and testosterone affect an enzyme called LPL. If these hormones are high, LPL is suppressed and less fat is pulled from our circulation and put into our fat cells. If they are low, more fat is pulled into the cells. When we exercise, LPL activity decreases on our fat cells and increases on muscle cells. This prompts the release of fat from the fat cells so we can use it in our muscle cells for fuel. We get a little leaner. When we are finished exercising, the situation reverses. Now LPL activity stops in the muscle cells and increases in the fat cells to restock them from what they lost during exercise. We get fatter again. We also get hungry because our muscles crave protein after a workout to restock and rebuild but our fat is restocking too. The rest of our body tries to compensate for this energy drain and our appetite increases and activity decreases. The more sedentary we are, the more chance/time the body has to restock. Remember the caveman.

Triglycerides are molecules made from 3 fatty acid molecules and 1 glycerol molecule. These fatty acids and glycerol molecules are small and they can go into our fat cells easily where they join to form the larger triglycerides. We need to break up these larger molecules to be able to burn them. Insulin makes you store these fatty acids that make triglycerides. Insulin uses the enzyme LPL to pull fat out of the blood into the cells. Insulin also can break up the triglycerides that are in our blood, and these smaller molecules can now go into the fat cells too. In men, LPL is more active generally in the fat cells of the gut (in women it's below the waist) but this activity is suppressed when there are enough male or female hormones. When our hormones are low, the LPL is more active and more fatty acids are deposited in those cells.

That is why we put on weight during and after male and female menopause.

There is another enzyme called HSL that breaks down triglycerides in the fat cells. Insulin suppresses this enzyme. Insulin also turns on a mechanism in fat cells to get them to pull glucose into themselves, which is another way to store fat/fuel. It also works to make more fat cells to store this extra glucose. Insulin does everything in can to increase storage of fat and to decrease the burning of it.

When we are stressed or when our insulin levels are high, an enzyme called cortisol is made. This enzyme puts fat into our cells. When insulin levels are low, cortisol burns fat. Insulin also works to keep protein stored away in muscles and not available for energy. As we fatten, our energy demand increases, just doing our daily movements, and we get hungry for more carbs that are more available than the protein stored in our muscles. These carbs cause insulin to be released and cortisol to put fat into our cells-talk about a vicious cycle.

The more carbs we eat, the more insulin is secreted, the more likely our cell and tissues will become resistant to it. The cells don't want more insulin because it it toxic to them. They make it harder for insulin to do its job to get the glucose out of the bloodstream. Our body is trying to keep blood sugar levels in check, so our pancreas makes more insulin that causes more insulin resistance in the cells - another vicious cycle! Type II diabetes occurs when the pancreas can no longer secrete enough insulin to compensate for the insulin resistance in the cells.

Fat, muscle, and liver cells don't become resistant at the same time or in the same way. If our muscle cells are sensitive (receptive) to insulin, they will take carbs and use them for energy - we will be lean and physically active. If they are insensitive, then fat cells will take the carbs and store fat - we will be fat and sedentary. As we get older, our different cells get more insulin resistant. This happens to muscles first so more carbs go to the fat cells that are still sensitive (receptive). Our metabolism slows because we are getting fat. As we age, the cells in the gut get sensitive sooner. Fat around our middles is caused by this and hormone levels becoming lower.

Genes control insulin secretion and sensitivity or insensitivity. Fat children are born to fat parents. The higher the levels of blood sugar in the mother, the higher the levels in the baby. Sometimes this doesn't show up till middle age. Mothers who gain excessive weight during pregnancy or who become diabetic during pregnancy have bigger babies.

Not all foods that have carbs are are equally fattening. The most fattening ones are the ones that have the most effect on your blood sugar/insulin levels such as those that we can digest quickly such as refined flour, bread, cereal, pasta, beer, fruit juices, sodas, potatoes, rice, corn, etc. These are also less expensive foods. This is one reason why the poor are fatter. The glycemic index tells us which carbs are better or worse. Some people are sensitive to any carbs-vegetables and fruits included. Sugars and high fructose corn syrup don't always have immediate effects but will cause problems in the long run. Sugars are worse than starchy carbs. That is why Africans and Asians are thin. They eat starchy (not refined) carbs but not sugars. The Japanese eat 1/4 the sugar and high fructose corn syrup the Americans do. The French eat 1/2 the Americans do. We have to become insulin resistant to develop the "Western" diseases. Thinking about eating carbs releases insulin that makes us hungry. We crave the foods that are the worst for us. Low fat products have more sugar added or carbs. In low fat yogurt, the fat is replaced with high fructose corn syrup.

Our total cholesterol is made up of: LDL that is called the "bad" cholesterol, HDL that is called the "good" cholesterol, and triglycerides. Cholesterol is good for the brain. Having low HDL puts us at a greater risk for heart attacks than having a high total or LDL cholesterol. In women, HDL levels are so good at predicting future heart disease that they are all the doctors look at. Carbs lower our HDL levels. There are large and small LDL proteins in our blood. LDL particles carry triglycerides and cholesterol around our blood. Small LDL particles work their way into the nooks and crannies in our arteries and cause plaque build up. The cholesterol is just along for the ride and not the problem. Carbs make LDL particles smaller. Eat less carbs and the LDLs particles get larger. High levels of triglycerides are also not good and can cause heart attacks and carbs elevate triglycerides. Eating a low fat diet may lower our LDL but it will raise our triglycerides.

The thought that saturated fat clogs arteries by raising cholesterol is a hangover from the science of 30-40 years ago. LDL and total cholesterol are the two risk factors most obviously modified by statin drugs. These drugs do prevent heart disease and save lives. So, the doctors reasoned, would a diet that lowered LDL and total cholesterol would do the same so a diet that did the opposite must be the cause of heart disease. Saturated fats raise total cholesterol and LDL so they must cause heart disease and diets that restrict these must prevent it. Because a drug lowers LDL and prevents heart disease does not necessarily imply that it prevents heart disease because in lowers LDL. Take aspirin, for example, it cures headaches and prevents heart disease. No one would say that aspirin prevents heart disease because it cures headaches. What drugs do and diets do are two entirely different things. Statin drugs - increase cancer risk because they lower critical levels of coQ10. The brain needs cholesterol. Impaired thinking is a common complication with statin drugs. A safer way to lower cholesterol is to take an extract of sugar cane wax called Poliosanol.

More than 1/4 of the U.S. population suffers from metabolic syndrome: as we get fatter, we loose control of our blood sugar, get high blood pressure, atherosclerosis, heart disease, stroke (caused by low HDL, high Triglycerides, small dense LDL), Alzheimer's, and most cancers.

Everyone looses weight differently because there are too many factors in the mix so there is no one size fits all solution. Some people can loose weight by simply eliminating sugars while others need to eliminate more types of carbs. Trying to reverse decades of eating carbs might take more than a few months or years. Vegetarians who eat leafy green vegetables, whole grains, beans are eating all carbs even though most of them have a low glycemic index and will have trouble loosing much weight. All they can do is make their carb choices lower on the index. Their health will get better but they won't get leaner.

The idea is to eat as strictly as you can. Not restricting the amount of food but the types of food. You don't want to feel hungry during your day. Once you have lost the weight you want to loose, you can try to add one carb food at a time and see what happens. If you gain weight again, stop and try some other one. Carbs are addictive (sugar can be as addictive as cocaine, heroine and nicotine) so be careful when you add that it doesn't snowball from once a week to every day. If you loose 2 lbs a week, that's 7,000 calories of your own fat that you burned for fuel. That is 1,000 calories each day you didn't have to eat so you are less hungry and have more energy. Exercise is good for toning your muscles, your cardiovascular system, and lungs but not necessary as part of a weight loss program.

High protein diets are toxic. You need to eat fats too because you are now burning the fat stored in your cells as well as the fat you eat instead of the glucose from carbs. In the first stage of weight loss, the daily protein amount in your diet should be about 20% and the rest vegetables, leafy greens, some dairy, and possibly some low carb fruit. Insulin signals your kidneys to reabsorb sodium and you retain water that raises your blood pressure. When the insulin is lowered because you are not eating carbs, you loose the water weight but you also loose potassium in the process. Make sure you get extra salt in some form. Another thing happens by restricting carbs: your blood pressure and blood sugar go down, so watch out for side effects especially if you are taking medications for either of these conditions. Do not eat low fat or "lite" products as they contain more sugar and starches. When reading labels, you should subtract the dietary fiber from the total carbs to get the net carbs number. Vegetables net carbs should be 5 or less per serving. Meats or condiments should be 1 or less. Watch out for sugar as it comes in many forms. Read the labels on products closely.

Alcohol is a special case and is metabolized in the liver. 80% of the calories from a shot of vodka go straight to the liver to be converted into a small amount of energy and a large molecule called citrate. The citrate then fuels the process that makes fatty acids out of glucose. So alcohol will increase the production of fat in the liver. It might also make us fat elsewhere. Whether you store these fats as fats or burn them depends on whether you eat or drink carbs with the alcohol, which is often the case.

Let's look at lard that is considered the worst fat possible to eat. 47% is monounsaturated fat-considered good and it raises HDL and lowers LDL (90% of this fat is the same oleic acid that is in olive oil). About 40% is saturated fat (but a third of this fat is stearic acid as in chocolate) and it raises HDL and has no effect on LDL. The remaining 13% is polyunsaturated fat that lowers LDL and has no effect on HDL. So 70% of the fat in lard will improve your cholesterol profile and the remaining 30% will raise your LDL but also raise your HDL. If you replace carbs with an equal amount of lard, you will reduce your risk of having a heart attack.

Foods to eat to stay below 20 carbs a day till you are at your target weight.

1. meat & poultry all you want to feel full: all types
2. all fish: use the Monterey Bay Aquarium good fish to eat list
3. shellfish: shrimp, scallops, crab, lobster (not mussels or clams)
4. whole organic eggs

Eat every day:

2C leafy greens
1C vegetables
artichokes, asparagus, broccoli, Brussel's sprouts, cauliflower, celery, cucumber, eggplant, green beans, jicama, leeks, mushrooms, okra, onions, peppers, snow peas, pumpkin, shallots, sprouts, sugar snap peas, summer squash, tomatoes, wax bean, zucchini

fats and oils and butter: all allowed
salad dressings: all kinds (just watch carb count) 1 to 2 grams
drinks: water, club soda, essence flavored seltzers (zero carbs), coffee

Eat in limited quantities:

cheese up to 4oz: hard cheeses, cream cheese, goat cheese, mozza-
rella, brie, blue, Swiss, cheddar, cottage cheese
cream: up to 4T (half & half is not as good as heavy, light, or sour
"cream")
mayonnaise: up to 4T
olives: up to 6
avocado: up to 1/2 of the fruit
lemon/lime juice: up to 4t
soy sauce: 4T (low carb brands)
snacks: pepperoni, ham, beef, turkey, deviled eggs, nuts

CHAPTER 2

YOUR HEALTH

Ladies Problems:

When women go to see their gynecologist or general practitioner (GP) with aches and pains, many times these doctors just dismiss these complaints and hand their patient a pill. Rarely does a doctor look at the causes of the problem. He usually just treats the symptoms by writing a prescription. We trust the FDA to protect us when it comes to these prescription drugs. They are supposed to test these drugs for safety as well as efficacy. More often than not, they use safety tests done by the pharmaceutical company who is trying to get that drug approved instead of their own FDA tests! How's that for the fox watching the hen house. One half of the FDA approximate 400 million dollar budget is paid by the pharmaceutical companies. You wonder how this started? Back in 1992, AIDS activists were hoping to speed up the approval rate by the FDA of new drugs to treat AIDS. There was an agreement made that the FDA would speed up its process in return for "user fees" from the drug industry. The FDA feels that efficacy is more important than safety. Vioxx was one example of this policy. Three out of five people who were involved with the approval of the drug had pharmaceutical company connections. Over 100,000 people died from taking Vioxx and many more were crippled or had other health problems.

Another problem with drugs is the relatively new phenomenon of direct marketing of prescription drugs to the public on TV and in magazines often times using celebrities or athletes to help them sell them. Only the USA and New Zealand allow this kind of marketing. Patients now arrive at their doctors office armed with name of the disease they think they have and the pill they think they need to cure it and demand to have it. Many doctors just write the prescription. WorldWatch.org states that the USA has 5% of the world's population but takes 50% of the world's drugs. There are over 1,200 lobbyists for drug companies in Washington D.C. There are even names for mental illnesses that are made up to sell a drug. The insurance companies need to have a name for a disease to assign a code number on their insurance forms to get reimbursed. Alternative medicine doctors are often ridiculed, harassed, and even brought up on charges by the medical establishment for daring to suggest these synthetic drugs are bad for you.

The bottom line: You have to be proactive when it comes to your own health.

Estrogen Replacement Therapy:

When women come to their doctor during menopause with hot flashes, etc, they are often prescribed ERT (estrogen replacement therapy). This treatment implies that menopause is caused by a decrease in estrogen. They prescribe a dosage of estrogen that is 20 times more potent than what was produced by the woman at the peak of her fertility. Premarin and the form of progesterone they prescribe are toxic to brain cells. Menopause is the exhaustion of the nerves that regulate the pituitary, and is caused by over exposure to estrogen. Estrogen is in our bodies but also in the food we eat: soy products, plants, all unsaturated oils, meats with synthetic estrogens, and environmental estrogens such as pesticides and fluoride. Estrogen is a fat-soluble female hormone produced in the ovaries. Two common forms of estrogen: estradiol and estrone are both tumorogenic (they cause tumors), carcinogenic (causes cancer), and cardiotoxic (toxic to the heart). A natural form called estriol protects the brain, especially against Alzheimer's, and does not cause breast cancer (kale also contains natural estrogen). The rate of estrogen production varies with some women producing nine times more estrogen than others. Women can secrete a substantial amount of estrogen regardless of menopause or hysterectomy including the removal of ovaries. This estrogen comes from the adrenal glands and many other tissues. Androgen, from the adrenals, converting to estrogen increases with aging in both men and women. These women who produce more estrogen are in greater danger of producing breast and uterine tumors, both benign and cancerous. There are also other sources of estrogen other than what women produce in their ovaries and other cells. This adds to the problem of excess estrogen levels in susceptible women. Among these sources are: birth control pills; commercial meat; milk, eggs and dairy foods containing synthetic estrogen; excessive consumption of estrogenic foods (wheat germ, yeast and yeast containing foods, beverages such as beer and wine). In addition, pesticides, soy product and unsaturated fatty acids are estrogenic, even though structurally, they don't look like the estrogen molecule.

Menopause:

Menopause is a progesterone deficiency condition, not an estrogen deficiency condition. As women age, less progesterone is produced in comparison to estrogen. What causes progesterone to fall with aging? The production of progesterone from cholesterol is dependent on adequate cholesterol, adequate thyroid function plus vitamin A and certain enzymes. Taking natural progesterone (not synthetic) reverses this effect. Women on ERT can wean themselves from it but there will be withdrawal symptoms because estrogen converts to a cocaine-like derivative. As she starts her new progesterone and pregnenolone therapy, theses symptoms will subside. Natural progesterone balances or neutralizes any excess or deficiency of any hormones in the body. Natural progesterone has the anti-aging effect of thickening and smoothing aged and atrophied skin by increasing pigment cell size and branching. It does not cause healthy, young skin to thicken. Progesterone balances excess estrogen, which causes skin to atrophy and become thinner: so much for estrogen-containing cosmetics. Progesterone keeps the blood sugar level up, excess estrogen lowers blood sugar, causes constipation, migraine headaches, edema, increased fat storage, and general malaise. Natural progesterone causes regression of breast tumors. PMS symptoms also result from a relative estrogen surplus and progesterone deficiency and the outcome of a thyroid deficiency. Progesterone and thyroid hormones work together to prevent most of the female complaints related to PMS. How is progesterone best absorbed? Dr. Peat, who has done a lifetime of research on progesterone, says it is best absorbed orally. Avoid synthetic progestin's especially Provera as it has the most toxic side effects according to Dr. Lee.

Pregnenolone:

Pregnenolone is an anti-aging steroid precursor and is made in the body from LDL cholesterol. We need some cholesterol for this process to take place so it is a bad idea to artificially inhibit the formation of cholesterol with drugs and synthetic foods. Dr. Peat calls it a brain steroid because the largest concentration is there. In our bodies, enzymes convert pregnenolone to either progesterone or DHEA, depending on the tissue and need. As we age, we loose pregnenolone and need to replace it. To get pregnenolone we need adequate amounts of LDL cholesterol plus other nutrients, including vitamin A, thyroid hormone and enzymes. Taking both natural progesterone and pregnenolone does not suppress your body's ability to also make more. Taking synthetic progesterone has toxic side effects not observed with its natural counterpart. Natural progesterone is strong medicine just like thyroid or insulin. It can fight the toxic effects of cortisol, estrogen and testosterone. The classic effects of toxic levels of cortisol include daytime euphoria, insomnia plus hot flashes at night, osteoporosis, brain aging, atrophying of the skin and other signs of premature aging. Peat believes that stress-induced elevation in cortisol/cortisone can even cause diabetes. Pregnenolone is an anti-aging food and can be compared to a food supplement such as a vitamin. Pregnenolone may help restore impaired memory, relieve the symptoms of anxiety and panic attacks, and has been used to treat rheumatoid arthritis.

Progesterone fights all of the effects of estrogen and cortisol and has other healing benefits, according to Peat. DHEA also has anti aging and anti-obesity properties. DHEA is manufactured by the adrenal glands from pregnenolone from birth and peaks during an individual's mid-twenties. It thereafter levels off with age. In men who have decreased testosterone production resulting in decreased libido, DHEA, which can convert to testosterone, boosts libido almost as well as the real thing. Progesterone can also help reverse osteoporosis. Problems with DHEA: If you have prostate cancer, you have to watch taking DHEA because it converts to testosterone which can make this cancer worse.

Hot flashes:

The worst hot flashes occur when your thyroid function is low with a high lifetime estrogen level. These women have night sweats and a pounding heart. Hot flashes usually increase at night because darkness exacerbates any stress that causes adrenalin and cortisol to rise and calming calcium to decrease. If you drink any kind of alcohol in the evening, the hot flashes will be worse as alcohol raises your sugar level and then it drops during the night. When your hormones are out of balance, the hypothalamus in your brain mistakenly signals the body to sweat, dialate your blood vessels, and speed up your heart rate. This chain reaction can also be set in motion by "triggers", the most common of which are stress and anxiety, caffeine, sugar in all its forms including alcohol, and even spicy foods. They decrease during the day as blood sugar rises. This situation can be worse during the winter because of fewer daylight hours. These women also cannot retain sodium, which is why many of these women crave salt and have edema (fluid retention). Sea salt is a natural diuretic and is essential for mobilizing blood sugar, which lowers adrenalin. Instead of eating salt, many patients are told to avoid salt and take a diuretic plus potassium. Use non-iodized sea salt as it contains 48 minerals and table salt contains only sodium chloride. Dr. Peat suggests a (sea salt) salty snack before bed to help keep blood sugar up and cortisol down as the night progresses. Pregnenolone, which is a precursor to progesterone, also lowers cortisol level. Folic acid is a B vitamin that can interact with various types of receptors in the brain and influence these thermoregulatory centers and help the hot flashes. Some people have trouble absorbing folic acid so they can take L-Methylfolate instead.

Compiler's note: I have taken one 400 mcg of vitamin B9 (folate or folic acid) pill before bedtime when I have had alcohol that evening and that has taken care of my hot flashes during that night.

Hysterectomy:

When menopause is created surgically within minutes, by a hysterectomy, many problems arise. The sudden shock of the surgery causes the remaining organs to try frantically to take over some of the functions of the ones that were removed. Estrogen therapy is often prescribed to alleviate these symptoms. This seems a bit strange since estrogen excess and or progesterone depletion is one of the primary causes of problems leading to the hysterectomy in the first place. Women who have had a hysterectomy need a while longer to balance their hormones sufficiently to end their hot flashes but it does happen in a few months. Dr. Ray Peat, PhD says it takes up to one year to recover from a hysterectomy and only about 5 percent are actually necessary (mainly due to cancer). 20 percent are due to sterilization. One reason used for this operation is fibroids yet only 3% to 7% per 1000 fibroids become cancerous.

Thyroid diseases:

The thyroid's hormones regulate vital body functions like breathing, heart rate, central and peripheral nervous systems, body weight, muscle strength, menstrual cycles, body temperature, cholesterol levels, and much more. Hyperthyroidism or high thyroid hormone levels can result in: anxiety, ir- ritability, moodiness, sweating, hand trembling, hair loss. Hypothyroidism or low thyroid hormones can result in: trouble sleeping, fatigue, difficulty concentrating, dry skin and hair, depression, sensitivity to cold, joint and muscle pains. Foods that are good for thyroid: fish, nuts, carrots, sweet potatoes, organic beef, zinc, magnesium, and tomatoes. Foods that are bad: cruciferous vegetables, strawberries, processed foods, fatty foods, caffeine, sugary foods, soy, peaches, and pears.

Osteoporosis:

The information in this section comes mainly from the work of Dr. Ray Peat and Dr. John Lee, M.D. Peat and Lee pioneered in gathering experimental data providing that progesterone, not estrogen, prevents and reverses osteoporosis. It has been claimed that estrogen prevents osteoporosis and the lack of estrogen causes it. The strongest argument for the use of estrogen to prevent osteoporosis is that it causes decreased excretion of calcium in the urine. Estrogen's effect in decreasing urinary calcium is merely a toxic effect of estrogen, causing it to deposit into the soft tissues instead of bone tissue. Why do we assume that it's going into bone tissue just because it's not coming out into the urine?

Osteoporosis means "holey" bones. Bone is a living tissue-mineralized cartilage that renews itself every two to seven years depending on the type. Two kinds of cells work to make new bone and dissolve old bone. Osteoblasts (with a B) are bone makers. They mineralize the cartilage and that makes the bones strong. Osteoclasts (with a C) make new bone tissue. They dissolve the aged bone tissue, leaving little spaces. The osteoblasts jump in and fill up these spaces with fresh new bone. Bone making requires a balanced pH and many nutrients such as calcium balanced with phosphorus and magnesium, vitamin D in its hormonal form; vitamins K, A, E, C; minerals such as boron, sodium, zinc, copper, organic silica and strontium, essential fatty acids; and the proper hormonal balance. When this delicate balance of pH, nutrients and hormones is disrupted, old bone is not replaced by new bone. This is osteoporosis. It is not uncommon for American women to have lost 30% of their bone mass by the time they reach menopause. It is not uncommon to see 50% bone loss in a 65 year old woman.

Doctors first though that the increased risk of osteoporosis in menopausal women was due to a decrease in estrogen, hence ERT became popular. They tested women five years prior and five years after menopause and found a decrease in estrogen and an increase in bone loss.

Had they tested progesterone levels, they would have seen a bigger drop in progesterone. Progesterone stimulates osteoblastic (bone making) activity and thyroid hormone stimulates both bone making and dissolving activity. Old bone must be dissolved in order to make room for new bone. Dr. Lee treated patients with progesterone therapy and over a three-year period, their bone density increased by 15.4%. His results were independent of age and estrogen therapy.

How do we get these nutrients to help with the menopausal symptoms and osteoporosis? Natural, whole, unprocessed, organic foods contain just about all the building materials required to build bones. All the minerals and vitamins you need may be found in whole fruits like blueberries, grass fed dairy, green leafy vegetables and broccoli, almond and coconut milk, eggs, whole grains, legumes, nuts like walnuts, salmon and sardines, seaweeds, seeds (chia, flax, pumpkin, sunflower). Many people eat processed foods, which have been stripped of their nutrients. They have no building materials with which to build their skeleton. Some foods worsen the chance of osteoporosis. These include high phosphorus foods such as soda pop and excessive consumption of yeast. Many people believe that animal protein, especially meat, can cause osteoporosis but, it's not the protein in the meat, it's the phosphorus, which must be balanced with calcium. In the United States, many people eat lots of meat and consume processed foods (refined sugars and carbohydrates), which have very little calcium. Excess sugar causes calcium loss and upsets the delicate ratio of calcium to phosphorus. In addition to estrogen, some of the other drugs that increase risk of osteoporosis include: Lasex (diuretic), fluoride (toxic to bones), and corticosteroids (anti-inflammatory drugs).

Bisphosphonates, a class of drugs used to prevent broken and deteriorating bones in cancer and osteoporosis patients, have been linked to a serious side effect called osteonecrosis, in which areas of bone in the jaw die. There are two varieties of the drugs, one taken intravenously by cancer patients (Zometa & Aredia), the other taken in lower-dose pill form by those with osteoporosis (Fosamax, Actonel, & Boniva). The incidence of osteonecrosis among cancer patients is estimated at between 1 and 10 percent, while incidences among osteoporosis patients is unknown.

Invasive dental procedures, such as tooth extractions, may spur osteonecrosis, so some dentists have stopped treating patients taking the drugs. These drugs stay in your bones for years, so no one knows how long the risk of osteonecrosis remains, even if the drug is no longer taken.

Weight bearing aerobic exercises and strength training are the primary ways to build bone. Things that are bad for calcium absorption: caffeine, wheat bran, spinach, sweet potatoes, rhubarb, sodium, meat, poultry, corn, and potatoes. Good for calcium absorption: Vitamin D, magnesium, taking calcium with orange juice, split your supplements throughout the day.

Osteoarthritis:

This is a very common arthritis among older people. It is a chronic condition of the joints. It happens when the protective cartilage on the ends of the bones wears down over time. Turmeric or curcumin is a very powerful anti inflammatory for your aches and pains. Use along with boswellia for joint and connective tissue support.

Lyme disease:

Lyme disease has becoming more and more common due to the increased deer population that exists side by side with suburbia. The deer carry the ticks and deposit them in our gardens, on our pets, and eventually into our homes. The ticks carry spirochete bacteria that stream into the body tissues. The symptoms of Lyme disease occur in three stages and may take several days to several weeks to start after the initial infection. Stage one: distinctive target shaped expanding rash that usually but not always develops a circular rash. Stage two: headache, muscle and joint pain, fever chills, fatigue, swollen lymph nodes, skin lesions. Stage three: meningitis, Bell's palsy, irregular heartbeat, Rheumatoid Arthritis. Osteoarthritis conditions: nerve numbness & tingling in hands and feet, memory lapse, mood swings, insomnia. Treatment of Lyme disease is usually a course of antibiotics. Increasing the circulation to help flush out the toxins built up from the infection can help too. Drink plenty of water. Using a far infrared sauna is also helpful as it stimulates the cells and activates the lymph system, which eliminates toxins from the body. Toxins are also eliminated from the body by the liver and kidneys. By detoxifying through the skin in the far infrared sauna, you lighten the burden on the liver and kidneys.

Headaches:
Headaches are caused by many factors both structural and physiological. They require physical and nutritional therapies plus recognition of dietary imbalances. Structural problems include TMJ (jaw joint problems), upper cervical (neck) problems, cranial problems, misaligned coccyx (tailbone), and physical trauma. When the spine is not correctly aligned and the head is bent downward the nerve supply to the head is compromised. Theses nerves also go through the stomach, gallbladder and pancreas. People with digestive or liver/gallbladder problems often develop headaches. Physiological and/or chemical imbalances are related to allergies and other health problems resulting from enzyme deficiencies like liver and gallbladder problems or hormonal problems such as hypothyroidism (low thyroid). A common hormonal cause of headaches in women, including migraines, is estrogen dominance, caused by hypothyroidism and aggravated by birth control pills or ERT.

Stress can cause tension headaches. There are many ways to relieve stress: mediation, chiropractic treatment, having massage therapy, taking a vacation and eliminating the cause of the stress like a stressful job or lifestyle.

The upper cervical headache is caused by the misalignment of the upper cervical vertebrae. People suffering from this problem can have many symptoms, not just severe headaches but dizziness, indigestion, severe constipation, problems with urination, sudden sinking spells, etc. Besides going to a chiropractor you can take an enzyme formula called Thera-zyme Sym for relief.

The coccyx headache occurs when the coccyx (tail bone) is misaligned. A neural sheath is attached to the coccyx and goes all the way from the tailbone to the brain. When the coccyx is misaligned many symptoms arise such as; migraines, sciatica, low back pain, and others. Both acupuncture and chiropractic treatments can realign the coccyx.

The migraine headache can also be caused by low blood sugar. If you remove refined sugar from your diet and take one of the Thera-zyme formulas, they will lessen.

The estrogen migraine is common in females who take birth control pills and who use estrogen as a morning after pill to prevent conception. They always occur in hypothyroid women who are estrogen dominant even though they don't take any form of estrogen therapy. This kind of headache is easy to diagnose because it occurs at ovulation and/or menses and subsides thereafter. This type of headache is often accompanied by vomiting, general malaise, and mood swings. There are always nutritional factors involved. The most common is excess sugar craving and/or consumption, excess consumption of chocolate. Natural progesterone therapy is always indicated, but low thyroid function is the cause because hypothyroid women cannot produce adequate progesterone. In addition, enzyme deficiencies, notably low blood sugar, must be properly diagnosed and corrected. Headaches can also be caused by a lack of magnesium.

Aging:

Aging diseases are associated with damaged DNA. Fluoride inhibits DNA repair. Melatonin protects the brain but it declines as we age. We make melatonin when we are sleeping and the maximum secretion happens from 10 pm for the next 8 hours. Adults need 7-8 hours of sleep. During sleep, tissue repair happens, human growth hormone is made, our immune system is strengthened, more sleep equals less risk of high blood pressure, heart disease, type 2 diabetes, weight gain. Curcumin (tumeric) is a very powerful antioxidant and it even helps make chemotherapy more effective.

Alzheimer's, Multiple Sclerosis, Parkinson's disease:

Alzheimer's, Parkinson's and strokes are partially caused by improper diet, not enough B-12, and not enough sleep. These neuromuscular diseases are all caused by inflammation in the brain and free radical activity. There are specific triggers for these two things. These triggers are: pesticides, herbicides, harmful ingredients in food and beverages, toxic metals in our air, water or food, various sugar substitutes, omega-6 fats such as; soybean, canola, sunflower, safflower, peanut, and corn oils, vaccines including flu shots which contain mercury, excitotoxins (mercury, aluminum, cadmium, and lead), nutritional deficiencies, hormonal imbalances, lack of exercise, or too much aerobic exercise. Excitotoxins cause specific neurons to burn out and die which causes neurological diseases. Excitotoxins also cause inflammation. Free radicals damage brain cells that eventually then die. Antioxidants neutralize free radicals and the antioxidant glutathione is a one good to take.

Avoid MSG (mono sodium glutamate) because glutamates take glutathione out of your body. MSG is still in many products but the manufacturers are using some different names for them. If you see anything listed on the label with the word glutamate in it, you are getting MSG just in a different form. Eating gluten free foods helps keep neurodegenerative diseases away.

Dementia is a type of Alzheimer's and not a separate disease. Keeping your overall cholesterol levels managed below 200 and eating more vegetables that have beta-carotene, vitamin C, and vitamin E can help. Do not eat a low fat diet because your brain needs some cholesterol, just not too much. Many people who are on a low cholesterol diet or are using statin drugs to lower their cholesterol for a period of time eventually develop Alzheimer's.

The best things that help people with Parkinson's are: NAC, luteolin, baicalein, curcumin, and quercetin. These all calm the microglia (the immune cells that play a central role in the disease). Coq10 in oil, acetyl-L-carnitine, B vitamins, the supplement pyruvate all increase brain energy production. Eventually a brain cell's function becomes impaired.

People with Alzheimer's and Parkinson's have chronic nutrient deficiencies long before the disease shows up. Many Alzheimer patients have elevated homocysteine levels. Homocysteine is a brain cell toxin that can excite brain cells to death. Vitamin E and C, antioxidants from plants all protect the brain from free radicals and excitotoxicity. Women have more Alzheimer's, Parkinson's, and dementia. This is because women loose their reproductive hormones faster and more than men. Testosterone is very protective of the brain but female hormones protect brain cells even more than testosterone. Choline (one of the B vitamins) is good for the brain and is in eggs, dairy, toasted wheat germ, peanut butter, almonds, oat bran, codfish, beef, turkey, and chicken. Foods that are good for your brain are: coconut oil, fish oil, eggs. Vitamins that are good: L-theamine, B vitamins, folic acid, choline, N-acetyl, acetyl L'carnitine, ginko biloba ashwagandha, and bacopa. Popular cold medicines like Tylenol PM, Benedryl, Claritin, Dimetapp, Zyrtec, etc. are dangerous for elderly people because they block acetylcholine that works in the brain to transmit electrical impulses between nerve cells. See the Source section for the name of a new good book on Alzheimer's.

Your Digestive System or Gut:

A healthy gut is important because it plays a 70% role in our immune system function. Due to the common problems of modern processed foods; soil depletion, exposure to toxins, and pesticides, over consumption of sugar and high levels of stress, you simply don't get enough of the probiotics your body needs. If you eat foods that you can't digest, they become toxins in your body and cause many health problems that you might not correlate with bad digestion: Acne, hives, rashes, colon problems, lung problems, constipation, diarrhea, bad breath, Parkinson's and so on. There is a connection between the health of your gut and neurodegenerative diseases.

If you have bacteria in your gut, there will be bacteria in your gums too which causes gum disease. Probiotics increase our good bacteria in the gut. They are especially good to take after a treatment of antibiotics as antibiotics kill your good bacteria along with the bad. Good sources: kombucha, Gouda cheese, sauerkraut, live culture plain flavor yogurt, tempeh, supplements. Buying a probiotic - things to consider: a brand that contains 25-50 billion probiotics per capsule with 5 or more strains. Prebiotics also need to be included in the formula. Packaging should protect the probiotics from light and heat.

Prebiotics are non-digestible dietary fiber that promotes and nourishes the growth and activity of good bacteria already in your gut. Coffee helps increase the growth of powerful anti-inflammatory probiotics. Eating whole foods and taking digestive enzymes to help digestion can solve these problems. Certain enzymes are usually deficient when female problems occur. Protease, the enzyme that digests protein, is very important in calcium metabolism. Many women who have PMS are protease deficient. In menopause, there is often a lipase enzyme deficiency. Lipase is used to digest fats. Many women benefit from taking extra protease and or lipase enzymes. Other things you can do: avoid MSG, get tested for gluten sensitivity, avoid inflammatory foods like high fructose corn syrup, omega 6 oils, supplements that contain iron, don't take vitamin C with meals because it increases iron absorption. Eat some grapefruit, take magnesium citrate or magnesium malate, glutathione.

There is a class of carbohydrates called FODMAPs that pull water into your intestinal tract. These foods may not be digested well and could be fermented upon by bacteria in the intestinal tract when eaten in excess. You have heard of beans and cabbage causing gas, bloating, cramping, and diarrhea. That is because they are only several examples of the FODMAPs. A low FODMAP diet can help IBS (irritable bowel syndrome). Eating FODMAPs can also hurt your weight loss chances as they make you retain water. There is a complete list of them on the Internet. Not all people are bothered by all of these foods. You need to go off as many as possible for at least a week and then add one at a time back to your diet to see if you get gas and bloating.

Indigestion:

Indigestion can manifest in the form of heartburn, reflux, bloating, gassiness and chest pain. The common assumption is that by taking the antacid, these symptoms will dissipate. It is assumed that too much acid is the cause of the problem. Acid production is required for adequate digestion. Without it, you do not breakdown your foods, especially proteins. When the acidity of the stomach gets too low, the food does not get digested and is passed into the small intestine undigested where it can putrefy and create gas or regurgitate as in reflux. Chronic stress and age reduce the production of acid in the stomach. You have to look at what may be inhibiting acid production. Eating too much, or too fast, eating high-fat foods, drinking too much alcohol or caffeinated beverages, taking drugs like aspirin or ibuprofen. Dairy products can cause problems in people who are allergic to them. Taking something like Tums only makes the problem worse by lowering the acids. Try plant based digestive enzymes instead. Different enzymes work on different types of foods. Eating more raw leafy greens and vegetables because they contain B vitamins that naturally help your body to make these enzymes.

Parasites:

Marcelle Pick started Women to Women in 1986 and over the years saw patients who were suffering from digestive problems like bloating, constipation, diarrhea, gas and fatigue. She often sent these patients to gastroenterologists who then diagnosed irritable bowel syndrome. They followed their diet and medication recommendations but, all too often, found no relief.

After a trip to Mexico, where she got "Montezuma's Revenge", she started to develop the same symptoms as her patients. She sent a stool sample to the lab but nothing showed up as abnormal. After asking around the alternative medicine community, she found another lab and this time the results came back showing parasites.

Now she tests every woman who comes to her with a diagnosis of IBS and 40% of them have intestinal parasites though many have never left the United States. Her expectation was that parasites only occur in third world countries. One key source is fruits and vegetables that are imported from third world countries. They don't have the regulations for sanitation that we have. Salad bars and the increase in dining out worsen the odds of getting parasites.

Other factors in the rise of intestinal parasite include the ease and frequency of worldwide travel, increased immigration, and contaminated water supplies. She believes environmental pollution plays a role by suppressing the immune system on a number of levels.

Any woman suffering from gastrointestinal upset should see their doctor. Tests need to be done to evaluate the flora of the intestines and to establish if there is a parasite infection, systemic yeast, and/or food sensitivity. With these tests results as a guide, the proper treatment can take place. There are many parasite cleanses available from your local health food store or natural doctor. Different parasites have also been linked with asthma, eczema, psoriasis, epilepsy, muscular dystrophy, cystic fibrosis, and even Down syndrome.

Uric acid problems:

Uric acid is a waste of protein metabolism. It is also present in large quantities in some foods. It causes problems because humans do not possess the enzyme to digest it to a soluble form. When uric acid precipitates, it can cause kidney stones or gout. Gout is a problem where uric acid crystals deposit in the joints, causing a painful inflammatory response.

How do uric acid stones form? Uric acid stones form if too much uric acid is present in the urine to remain dissolved. They form quickly as there are no known inhibitors in human urine to cope with this fluctuation in output. A sudden uric acid load from food can also precipitate a new stone. This means that what you eat and drink directly affects your chance of developing stones.

To help prevent a problem, drink enough water daily. This keeps the urine more consistent in pH. Drinking water is so effective that you can actually dissolve stones that have already formed. Also, watch the acid in your diet and various foods that have a concentration of uric acid. Some foods that are high in uric acid: shellfish, organ meats, any red meat, game, peas, beans, anchovies, mackerel, sardines and herring.

Uric acid's solubility in urine is dependent on the pH, or acidity of the urine. At a pH of 7 (neutral), urine can dissolve 1000 times the amount of uric acid than at pH5 (acidic). Most people who form frequent uric acid stones have acidic urine. Urine becomes acidic in response to diet. Proteins are the greatest source of acid in the diet. After a meal high in protein, conditions become ideal for stone formation. Avoid eating large portions of meat at one sitting and drink plenty of fluids (but not water…drink wine or beer) <u>with</u> your meal. Adding some foods that have an anti-acid effect into a meal can also help. Alcohol, especially in binges can cause an attack of gout or kidney stones. The effect of alcohol is to cause dehydration, which then increases the risk of uric acid buildup - especially if consumed in more than moderate volumes.

Type II diabetes:

A diagnosis of type II diabetes is often a grim precursor to heart disease, kidney failure, stroke, nervous system damage, and other life–threatening complications. It often affects people with high blood pressure and bad cholesterol numbers. Diabetics have 10 times more insulin than normal in their bodies. Insulin makes you store fat and causes weight gain. Many of the 20 million Americans suffering from diabetes could dramatically improve their condition, not just "manage" it as most treatment programs aim to do.

One nutritional approach is a low fat vegan diet that can help many patients cut their blood sugars, improve their insulin sensitivity, and reduce, if not eliminate, their medications. Rather than compensate for malfunctioning insulin, like other treatments, the diet actually helps an individual's own insulin work better by altering what goes on inside that person's cells. The diet lowers cholesterol and high blood pressure, helps weight loss, and improves energy. There is no cutting of calories, portion control, or limiting of carbohydrates. If you do not want to restrict yourself this much, you can also do a low carbohydrate diet.

Heart disease:

People are misled to believe that if their cholesterol levels are normal they are at low risk for heart attacks and strokes. If this is true, then why do half the people who suffer heart attacks have normal cholesterol? The cause of heart disease is inflammation of the artery walls. Cholesterol will not clog your arteries if there is nowhere for it to attach like a ridge in the inflamed arterial wall. Statin drugs that lower cholesterol don't address this problem. Elevated homocysteine levels, in the blood, damages the wall of the artery. We call this process arteriosclerosis. Too much homocysteine in your blood literally shreds your arteries from the inside out. B vitamins can help reduce homocysteine levels in your blood. Insulin resistance in type II diabetes is one of the major causes of elevated cholesterol levels, inflammation of the arteries, and higher blood pressure. Another important risk factor in heart disease is low thyroid function. Men have one more factor to consider, low free testosterone that can predict the severity of artery blockages. Adequate cholesterol levels are required in order for the body to make testosterone. A man on statins may not have enough cholesterol to make testosterone thus increasing the risk of heart attack or stroke! Optimal free testosterone levels are 150-210.

Our total cholesterol is made up of: LDL that is called "bad" cholesterol, HDL that is called the "good" cholesterol, and triglycerides. Cholesterol is good for the brain. Current thinking suggests having a total cholesterol level of 200-240 may actually be good for your brain. Having low HDL puts us at a greater risk for heart attacks than having high total or LDL cholesterol. In women, HDL levels are so good a predicting future heart disease that they are all the doctors look at. Carbs lower our HDL levels. There are large and small LDL proteins in our blood. LDL particles carry triglycerides and cholesterol around our blood. Small LDL particles work their way into the nooks and crannies in our arteries and cause plaque build up. The cholesterol is just along for the ride and not the problem. Carbs make LDL particles smaller. Eat less carbs and the LDLs particles get larger. High levels of triglycerides are not good either and can cause heart attacks and carbs elevate triglycerides. Eating a low fat diet may lower our LDL but it will raise our triglycerides because they usually have more sugar in them.

The thought that saturated fat clogs arteries by raising cholesterol is a hangover from the science of 30-40 years ago. LDL and total cholesterol are the two risk factors most obviously modified by statin drugs. These drugs do prevent heart disease and save lives. So, the doctors reasoned, that a diet that lowered LDL and total cholesterol would do the same and a diet that did the opposite must be the cause of heart disease. Saturated fats raise total cholesterol and LDL so they must cause heart disease and diets that restrict these must prevent it. Because a drug lowers LDL and prevents heart disease does not necessarily imply that it prevents heart disease because in lowers LDL. Take aspirin, for example, it cures headaches and prevents heart disease. No one would say that aspirin prevents heart disease because it cures headaches. What drugs do and diets do are two entirely different things. Statin drugs increase cancer risk because they lower critical levels of coQ10. The brain needs cholesterol. Impaired thinking is a common complication with statin drugs. A safer way to lower cholesterol is to take an extract of sugar cane wax called Policosanol. Dr. Andrew Weil M.D. and others say that another way to help is to eat foods that contain coQ10 or take the supplement coQ10 that is an antioxidant that is made in the body. Not everyone makes enough of this enzyme that generates energy in cells. It generates the most energy in the kidneys, liver, and heart. It helps with oxygen utilization and energy production in the heart muscle cells. It helps with LDL cholesterol, circulatory health, and supports heart muscles and vessel walls.

Heart Attack - Coumadin and Vitamin K interaction:

Warfarin (Coumadin) is a medicine prescribed for people at increased risk of forming blood clots. Some medical conditions make the blood clot too easily and quickly. This can cause serious health problems because clots can block the flow of blood to the heart or brain. Coumadin can prevent harmful clots from forming. Blood clots are formed through a series of chemical reactions in your body. Vitamin K is essential for those reactions. Coumadin works by decreasing the activity of Vitamin K. To help Coumadin work effectively, it is important to keep your Vitamin K intake as consistent as possible. To help make it easier to keep your intake of Vitamin K consistent you should limit your intake of "high" Vitamin K to 1 serving a day, limit "moderately high" foods to no more than 3 servings a day. You should report any significant changes to your diet or weight to your doctor. Foods that are "high" in Vitamin K are kale, spinach (cooked), turnip greens, collards, Swiss chard, parsley, and mustard greens. Eat no more than 1/2cup per day. Foods that are "moderately high" in Vitamin K. Brussels sprouts, spinach (raw), turnip greens, green leaf lettuce, broccoli, endive, romaine. Eat no more than 1 cup per day. Alcohol, dietary supplements, Vitamin E, and antibiotics can also be a problem so check with your doctor.

Stroke and homocysteine:

If your homocysteine is too high, there are problems with inflammation in your body and with the utilization of B vitamins. High levels of it can also affect bone density. If it's too low it can affect memory, energy, and mood. According to a 2005 study, people genetically prone to high concentrations of homocysteine have a higher risk of stroke than other individuals. Establishing homocysteine, an amino acid in the blood, as the cause of

stroke is important for the vitamin and supplements industry as there is evidence that folic acid and B vitamins can lower its concentration, therefore
protecting heart health. Stroke is the third most common cause of death
in developed countries. Smoking and socioeconomic class (bad diet) also
increases homocysteine concentrations and stroke risks which confounds
the study results.

Tips to prevent strokes: maintain a healthy diet by eating less red meat,
eating more vegetables and berries, coconut oil and olive oil. Stay hydrated,
exercise regularly, get restful sleep, take nutritional supplements, avoid pro-
long stress.

Breast cancer:

John Robbins writes that, in 1991, breast cancer developed in 1 out of 9
American women and it caused 32% (175,000 diagnoses) of all cancers
in women. Ovarian cancer was 20,500 diagnoses and 12,400 were ex-
pected to die. (Sources: National Institutes of Health, Centers for Disease
Control, American Medical Assoc. and others) In 1998, the National
Cancer Institute announced that there had been a breakthrough in the
prevention of breast cancer. A new drug called Tamoxifen had cut the rate
of new breast cancer by 45% in a study of 13,400 women. Unfortunately,
the acclaim was a bit premature as later data showed only 17 out of 1,000
women avoided breast cancer after taking the drug for 5 years and 12 of
them developed uterine cancers and 10 potentially fatal blood clots! Using
this toxic drug is a strange way to prevent cancer. Zeneca Pharmaceuticals,
that sells Tamoxifen under the name Nolvadex has spent a lot of money
promoting this drug that costs more than $1,000 per year (in year 2001
$'s) that translates to billions in annual sale possibilities. Zeneca is also the
company that sponsors the Breast Cancer Awareness month whose focus is
on educating women about early detection like mammograms. This seems
wonderful but by the time a cancer can be detected on a mammogram, it
already exists so it is already too late to prevent! Many people believe this

misplaced focus on mammograms is diverting the publics' attention away from real prevention possibilities. There is another problem. The parent company of Zeneca is a company called Imperial Chemical Industries (ICI) that is one of the world's largest manufacturers of pesticides and plastics and one of the world's most notorious chemical polluters. They earn more than $300 million a year from sales of a carcinogenic herbicide Acetochlor while simultaneously marketing Tamoxifen that is now the world's bestselling cancer therapy drug. Sadly, there is not a word in the literature associated with BCAM (Breast Cancer Awareness Month) to suggest the role diet can play in cancer prevention, nor any mention of how to decrease other forms of exposure to carcinogens.

Mammograms and breast cancer:

Mammograms involve radiation and do not detect tumors/cancer as early as the relative newer procedure called a thermal imaging system or thermography. About 15% of all breast cancer diagnosis's are in women under 45 year of age. Breast cancer in young women is more aggressive and they have poorer survival rates. Thermography is quick and easy and more comfortable and involves no radiation and is more accurate under the age of 50. If you are over fifty, it is good to do both because they pick up different problems.

Genetics:

Your genetics are not a death sentence for some diseases, just a predisposition for that disease. Whether the disease is expressed or not depends on other factors such as your eating habits, toxins in your environment, stress, etc. Only 2% of all breast cancers are genetic.

CHAPTER 3

IT IS MORE THAN JUST PAMPERING

Reflexology:

This is a natural healing art based on the principle that there are places in the feet, hands, and ears that correspond to every part, gland and organ in your body. Putting pressure on these places, a reflexologist can relieve tension, improve circulation and help promote the natural function of the related areas of the body. Once again you are getting energy to flow to the area of the problem.

Yoga:

Yoga is a combination of breathing and stretching, balance, and strengthening exercises. It has been practiced for centuries in India and other "Eastern" countries and is a very relaxing and meditative practice.

Meditation:

An ancient Eastern practice that is actually becoming popular in the Western world among people from all walks of life. Anyone can use meditation to help them cope with medical problems, stress, and anxiety by way of thought, contemplation, and reflection. There are various types of meditation such as transcendental, Zen, Taoist, Buddhist, etc. But they all hold to the basic principles of consideration and quiet thought. The end goal of all types of meditation lead to a mind that is quieted and free from stress by the use of quiet contemplation and reflection. There are a variety of benefits from regular meditation. Physical benefits include a decrease in blood pressure, an improvement in breathing, and your resting heart rate is lower which takes some of the stress off the heart. It can promote youthful skin and appearance. Psychologically, meditation can also improve your moods, memory, and lessen depression.

Jin Shin Jitsu:

It is the very ancient Japanese physio-philosophy art of releasing tensions that are causes for various symptoms in the body. In the 1950s', this technique was brought to the U.S. by a lady named Mary Burmeister. She, in turn, has taught many other practitioners. Our bodies contain several energy pathways that feed into all of our cells. When one or more of these pathways become blocked, this damming effect may lead to discomfort or even pain. This blockage or stagnation will not only disrupt the local area, but will continue and eventually disturb the paths of energy flow throughout the body. Having a session is very relaxing. You lie on a padded massage table and the practitioner holds various pressure points to release the blockages and restore the energy flow throughout your body.

Reiki:

This is a Japanese technique for stress reduction and relaxation that also promotes healing. The technique uses the "laying on of hands" to get our "life force energy" flowing through our body. If this energy is low, we are more prone to sickness and stress. A treatment feels like a wonderful glowing radiance that flows through you. Reiki treats the whole person. It also works in conjunction with all other medical and therapeutic techniques to relieve side effects and promote recovery. During a Reiki class, this simple technique is transferred by the Reiki master to the student. Now the student can perform the technique at home.

Therapeutic massage:

It is a type of deep tissue massage that is meant to have a therapeutic benefit on your body. It differs from relaxation message that is performed to help someone relax. Therapeutic massage can also be relaxing but it does more. It helps loosen muscles, improve muscle tone, and increase flexibility. It can be used in conjunction with physical therapy, wound care, cancer care and a variety of other treatments because it helps blood flow to the troubled area. Psychotherapists also use this massage as part of their treatment program to alleviate severe depression, promote relaxation and increase trust. Someone who is able to do this type of massage has special training and has to be licensed by the state.

Foot Facts:

Twenty five percent of all the bones in your body are in your feet. If these bones get out of alignment so will the rest of your body. The pressure on your feet when running is as much as four times the weight of your body. The average woman walks 3 miles more per day than the average male. Women experience foot problems more than men. Walking is the best exercise for your feet. Standing in one spot is more tiring than moving because the same few muscles are working all the time. Planter fasciitis is the inflammation of a thick band of tissue that connects the heal bone to the toes.

CHAPTER 4

TOXINS

We live in a toxic world. Before WWII, when chemicals started to become mass produced, there were no such things as SIDS (sudden infant death syndrome), chronic fatigue syndrome or ADD (attention deficit disorder). Our bodies have become virtual dumping grounds for the hundreds of thousands of toxic compounds that invade our air, water, and even the soil that nurtures our food.

More than 77,000 chemicals are in active production in North America. More than 3,000 chemicals are added to our food supply; and more than 10,000 chemicals in the form of solvents, emulsifiers, and preservatives are used in food processing, packaging, wrapping and storage.

Every day, all of us ingest tiny amounts of these chemicals. The EPA estimates there are more than 20,000 chemicals that our bodies cannot metabolize. Chemicals not metabolized are stored in the fat cells throughout our bodies where they continue to accumulate. As these chemicals build up, they alter our metabolism, cause enzyme dysfunction and nutritional deficiencies, create hormonal imbalances, damage brain chemistry, and cause cancer. Because the chemicals accumulate in different parts of the body and at different rates and in different combinations, there are a disturbingly large variety of different chronic illnesses that can result.

It is becoming apparent that the more we pollute our air, water, and food, we are also seeing an increase in disease. We must educate ourselves as to what is harmful to us and to our families and then avoid these things. There are also natural toxins like heavy metals, radon, plants, and pollens. We cannot control our exposure to all of these things but we can be aware that they exist. Microbial toxins like bacteria, yeast, mold, fungus, viruses, and parasites, that we are all exposed to, are best combated by building a healthy immune system through diet, supplementation and detoxification.

Air toxic sources:

Nuclear power plants release radioactivity in small amounts regularly into our air, water, and soil and this permissible activity is allowed by federal regulations. This doesn't mean it is safe. As they age, the potential for leaks also increases. Accidental releases are not always verified or documented.

Plastics in the home and office environment continually outgas into the air we breath. Think of all the smells in the air around you. Some are coming from the chemicals in plastics and are making their way into your bloodstream and eventually into all your organs. We breath in all kinds of pollution from auto exhaust to industrial and municipal incinerators

Microwave radiation transmitted from cell phones, computers screens, i pads, and TVs puts radiation in your body which causes problems in the brain, kills sperm, female eggs, and the use by mothers during pregnancy can even become a contributing factor to autism in her children.

Water toxic sources:

Runoff occurs naturally as soil is eroded and carried to various bodies of water. Toxic chemicals enter waterways through natural processes, such as volcanic eruptions, mud slides, forest fires. Runoff from human activity comes from point source places like sewage treatment plants, factories, or even homes. Regulations determine what type and what amount industries are allowed to release. These regulations vary by region, state, and nation. There is also "non point" source pollution where runoff does not go directly into but gets into the ground water. Non point sources of runoff can be large urban, suburban, or rural areas.

Household toxic sources:

Our homes can be more toxic that the outdoor air even in heavily polluted areas like Los Angeles and New Jersey. The following is a list of some of the chemicals found in our home with some of the negative effects.

1. Ammonia found in cleaners, disinfectants, fabric softeners, furniture polish can cause irritation to the eyes and respiratory tract.
2. Ethanol found in cleaners, disinfectants, mouthwash, sunscreens, and personal care products. Ethanol can cause central nervous system depression, vertigo, drowsiness, and more.
3. Formaldehyde found in mold & mildew cleaners, particleboard, carpets, many adhesives, paints, cleaning products, and personal care products. Inhaling the fumes can irritate the eyes, lungs, esophagus, and cause cancer. "Formaldehyde" has 50 different synonyms (as do many toxic chemicals) that chemical manufacturers use to disguise them in their products.
4. Nitrobenzene found in furniture polish can cause cancer, birth defects, heart, liver, and central nervous system damage.
5. Creosol found in cleaning products, disinfectants, paint removers, and personal care products can affect the central nervous system, cause depression, hyperactivity and irritability.
6. Phenol found in air fresheners, disinfectants, paint removers, furniture polish and many personal care products is linked to cancer, respiratory damage, respiratory arrest, and more.
7. Styrofoam products are made from polystyrene. The styrene in these containers migrates into your food or drinks. The higher the fat content of the food, and the hotter the drink, the more styrene that migrates. Don't forget the styrofoam trays that meat and vegetables come on in the market. Styrene mimics estrogen in the body and can therefore disrupt normal hormone functions. Styrofoam also never breaks down in the garbage stream so is a very serious environmental problem.

Avoid using "dry cleaning" to clean your clothes. These harsh chemicals can get on your skin and then into your body. If you must use dry cleaning, air the clothes out in the fresh air for several hours to get some of the chemicals to dissipate.

Avoid strong chemical household cleaners such as liquid detergents, disinfectants, toilet bowl sanitizers, pesticides, and insecticides. For a list of alternative remedies for pesticides and insecticides, go to www.panna. org. To clean, use environmentally friendly products or try white vinegar for counters and floors and a paste of baking soda and water for scrubbing power.

Do not microwave foods or liquids in plastic containers made with PVC's or polystyrene. Use Pyrex type glass if you have to microwave.

Avoid preparing foods in scratched Teflon coated pots and pans as the underlying aluminum is toxic. The new enamel lined pans are better.

Sunscreen lotions - chemicals in them cause cell damage. They need to be used correctly or they cause more damage than good. The better way to be out in the sun is to wear SPF 30 clothing and covering up during the middle of the day (10 am - 2 pm).

Cosmetics - many toxic chemicals are not listed in ingredients and are absorbed through skin and inhaled. Dark hair dyes have been found to cause cancer in laboratory animals. Some colors of nail polish have the toxin toluene in them, which is similar to benzene. Hair care products, lotions, after shaves, deodorants, mouthwashes and toothpastes all have ethylene glycol in them which is use in industry to break down protein and cellular structure (what skin is made of). Baby lotions, baby oil, Vaseline, lip products all contain mineral oil which clogs the pores hindering the skins ability to eliminate toxins, causing skin disorders. The use of lip balms interferes with the body's own natural moisturizing mechanism and creates chapped lips. Synthetic fragrances that are made from as many as 200 chemicals that are not listed on the labels in many personal care products can cause problems like asthma, headaches, rashes, and migraines. Many different personal care products, including perfume, also contain phthalates that are toxic and can cause liver or kidney damage and have adverse effects on reproduction.

Food related toxic sources:

About 10 billion land animals in the United States are raised for dairy, meat, and eggs each year. Factory farms account for 37% of methane emissions which has 20 time the global warming potential of CO_2. Manure can also contain traces of salt and heavy metals, which can end up in bodies of water where it accumulates in the sediment, concentrating as they move up the food chain. When manure is repeatedly over applied to farm land, it causes dangerous levels of phosphorus and nitrogen in the water supply. In such excessive amounts, nitrogen robs water of oxygen and destroys aquatic life. Heavy metals are resistant to degradation and therefore have persisted for many years in the environment. They build up in the food chain and are stored in the body fat of animals and humans. Human body fat now also contains more than 100 industrial chemicals. PCB contamination from historic uses and dumping is widespread though out the U.S. and the world. Disposal into the waterways has caused contamination of rivers, oceans, soils and even the polar ice cap. Many forms of wildlife have become contaminated with PCB's including fish and even polar bear meat.

Mercury contaminates fresh and saltwater fish (especially swordfish, tuna) and to a lesser extent, bottom dwelling shellfish and fish (lobster, crabs, clams, oysters, flounder). If you get a flu vaccine yearly, you increase your chance of getting Alzheimer's. There is mercury in flu vaccines. Mercury poisons critical brain enzymes. Luckily, there are flu vaccines available without mercury. Glutathione is a very powerful antioxidant that protects cells from mercury poisoning. Sweating can help get the mercury out of your body.

BPA is in the can linings of soups, sodas, vegetables, and even infant formula. It's also in some types of plastic bottles. BPA has been shown to cause birth defects.

Cadmium, aluminum, mercury, lead, and arsenic are some of the heavy metals added to the food chain from upstream industrial discharges, pesticide runoff, incinerator emissions, manufacturing smokestacks, as well as from aviation and auto exhausts.

Aluminum has also been considered suspect in contracting Alzheimer's, Parkinson's, and dementia by increasing brain levels of glutamate. Several products increase the absorption of aluminum and increase its toxicity in the brain. Fluoride and aluminum are added to municipal drinking water. MSG increases aluminum absorption.

The many chemicals used in food growing, harvesting, preserving, processing, preparation, cooking, and packaging may be invisible, but they are nevertheless present and end up stuck in our bodies. John Robbins points out that genetically engineered soy and corn that has been sprayed with Roundup - turns up in infant formula (soy), Doritos, Tostitos, and Fritos (corn) to name a few.

Mother's milk can have many toxins from the mother's body. So it is a good idea for the mother to detox as much as possible before getting pregnant even if she is not planning to nurse her baby. Most babies are born with many industrial chemicals even before the mother has a chance to nurse them.

Phthalates are in outgases from plastic wrap, Styrofoam, plastic bottles and other plastics. They are even in breast milk because of the mother's exposure. They can damage our hormone receptors that pick up hormone signals and tell cells to grow. If there is a cancer cell there, it will grow. The most common cancers these days are hormone related cancers like breast, testicular, and prostate.

Dioxins are created in part through the manufacture of plastics, pesticides and other chemicals and are rained on the soil that grows our food by air pollution. They are one of the most potent causes of cancer.

Once these toxins have built up in our bodies it is hard to get rid of them. As we get older, we see nothing suspicious about getting cancers, auto-immune diseases like lupus, arteriosclerosis, high blood pressure, arrhythmia, heart attack, rheumatoid arthritis, thyroiditis, high cholesterol, diabetes, colitis, allergies, Parkinson's disease, benign prostatic hypertrophy (prostate enlarges and constricts the flow of urine), multiple sclerosis, osteoporosis, heart failure, worn out joints requiring replacements, and other degenerative diseases in midlife.

Environmental causes of breast cancer:

There is evidence that breast cancer in females, testicular cancer, genital abnormalities, and reduced sperm counts in males is directly connected to the rise of chemical pollution on earth.

In 1992, Greenpeace released a study linking the increase in breast cancer worldwide to certain synthetic chemicals. Among their findings: industrial nations with more severe pollution have higher breast cancer rates than non-industrial nations, the correlation of animal fat intake with cancer may only be an indicator that chemicals persist in the animal fat, there is a parallel between the increase of breasts cancer and the use of synthetic chemicals. Airplanes, buses, restaurants, grocery stores, etc. are routinely sprayed with pesticides

The January 2006 report, State of the Evidence: What is the Connection Between the Environment and Breast Cancer? (www.breast-cancerfund.org), summarizing more that 350 recent studies in breast cancer research, cites exposure to radiation and synthetic chemicals as possible causes. Environmental factors that the report cites include xeno-estrogens (hormone disrupters) found in pesticides, fuels, plastic, detergents, and prescription drugs; solvents; hormones used in oral contraceptives and replacement therapy; ionizing radiation; aromatic amines from diesel exhaust, tobacco smoke, and grilled meats, and air pollutant created by internal combustion engines.

In 1961, one in 20 women got breast cancer. By 1994, one in 8 got it and the rate has stayed the same since for getting some form of breast cancer. Breast cancer is the second-leading cause of cancer deaths in women, exceeded only by lung cancer. It is the leading cause of cancer deaths among women 40-55. Yet less than one out of ten women diagnosed with breast cancer has a genetic predisposition.

Estrogen is a carcinogen unless opposed by or balanced by progesterone. Both men and women produce estrogen. Chemicals that mimic estrogen are called xeno-estrogens. Some xeno-estrogens that we are exposed to are: insecticides; petroleum byproducts such as PCB's; PVC, a very common plastic; dioxin, a byproduct from paper bleaching; herbicides, synthetic estrogens, such as DES; certain combustion products, from the incineration of trash.

Phytoestrogens are natural substances in certain plants that have estrogenic activity. Some of these include yeast, and certain herbs such as black cohosh, sage, and pennyroyal and the isoflavones in soy. These phytoestrogens are weaker because they must be digested, absorbed and assimilated before they can affect the body. Not so with xeno-estrogens.

Dr. Servan-Schreiber states that, even in the face of mounting evidence linking pesticides to cancer, U.S. pesticide use is on the rise. DDT has been banned in the U.S. since 1972 but is still used in many countries including Mexico. Before 1972, DDT was common in meat and dairy products. Because it is stored in our fat cells for decades, most Americans still carry residues. Endosulfan, a pesticide that was banned in 2012 in the U.S. (but still used in India and China), has estrogenic properties comparable to DDT. Endosulfan was found to be the 7th most commonly detected pesticide residue in food samples taken by the U.S. F.D.A. between 1986 and 1991. It was also detected in ground water in California, Maine, and Virginia.

Magnetic fields can boost the concentration of estrogens circulating in the blood. Magnetic fields, even those of low frequency, emanate from all electronic devices including TV's, computer display terminals, clocks, radios, and all battery-operated devices, including toothbrushes and toys.

CHAPTER 5

DETOXING YOUR LIFE

Before you start detoxing, you need to know what toxin is causing the problem so you can detox more efficiently. You can detox only so fast. Every body has its own rate and you can't rush it. As the body cleanses itself, there will be side effects. You need to help and strengthen your kidneys and liver before you start detoxing.

Detoxing ourselves:

Choosing more organic hair products, bath soaps, laundry detergents, perfumes, deodorants, etc. will help.

Sweating is a good way to remove mercury, pesticides, herbicides, and other toxic chemicals. Think far infrared sauna. Far infrared (FIR) waves are a safe form of light energy that is thermal. The human body can easily absorb far-infrared heat that actually goes 2-3 inches deep into muscular tissue and ligaments. This thermal effect within the deep layers of tissues improves blood circulation and promotes healing and wellness. Far infrared heat is widely used in the healthcare industry. As an example, babies are kept warm in their incubators by far infrared heat. The benefits of (FIR) are many: pain relief, reduces stress, improves blood circulation, removes harmful toxins and improves the immune system. This heat stimulates dilation of your blood vessels, which speeds the healing of sprains and strains, thus relieving pain and speeding the recovery time. It reduces stress by loosening the muscles and relaxing them in an overall massaging effect, soothing jagged nerves and knotted muscles. When toxins are present, blood circulation is blocked and cellular energy function is inhibited, which makes it difficult to fight disease. By increasing the blood circulation and lymphatic flow, the FIR heat can break down these materials and gases, encapsulate them and release them through perspiration. Daily sweating can help detoxify the body of carcinogenic heavy metals. FIR heat raises your inner body temperature, which strengthens and accelerates the immune system. An Amethyst Bed (or Bio Mat) works similarly to FIR but you lie on the bed instead of sitting in a big sauna style box. There are also many types of detox regimes that use chelation, special supplements, or a 10 day program of diet with pills and powder drinks such as Clear Change by Metagenics.

Detoxing our home:

Try reading labels and using simpler products for cleaning, etc. Avoid, as best you can, the chemicals mentioned in the last chapter. Open your windows and let the fresh air circulate around your house. The outside air may be polluted but that air is usually better than the inside air.

Detoxing our food:

Eat all organic fruits and vegetables if possible but some are more important to eat organically than others. The Environmental Working Group (EWR) has listed them as follows: **"The dirty dozen"** include: apples, blueberries, nectarines, peaches, strawberries, grapes, potatoes, kale, collards, spinach, sweet bell peppers, celery, and lettuce (due to pesticide spraying). Coffee and wine should also be organic too. **"The clean fifteen"** include: onions, sweet corn, avocado, asparagus, eggplant, mushrooms, cabbage, sweet peas, sweet potatoes, mango, pineapple, cantaloupe, watermelon, grapefruit, and kiwi. For organic meat, poultry, and eggs the animals need to be free ranging and fed 100% organic feed and not given any antibiotics or hormones.

CHAPTER 6

USE IT OR LOOSE IT!

Use it or loose it is so true. You have to move around to keep your muscles strong, get your circulation going, and work your cardiovascular system, etc.

Anything will help but the best and easiest exercises to try are walking, biking, and swimming. These are great choices because you need no real special equipment. If you pick swimming, try to stay out of a heavily chlorinated pool. There are many saltwater pools (including public pools) now that don't use this strong toxic chemical. Get off the couch and walk up and down the stairs a few extra times. No stairs! There are tiny portable stair masters that can do the job. Speaking of the couch, there are lots of exercise programs on cable or satellite TV and exercise DVD's to watch. Join a gym or the Y and do your own routine or join a class. Adding some light hand weights to your routine will help keep your bones strong. This will ramp up your BMR (basal metabolic rate) to burn more calories. A weight workout raises your BMR for 30 hours. A single hour cardio set raises it for only 4 hours. Think about working with a personal trainer. They can help you with a regime that fits your capabilities, health status, and schedule. Many gyms have them on staff. Recruit your best friend with whom to workout.

Another new way to get a good, efficient, and not strenuous workout in a short time is by using a machine called a power plate. They are found in some gyms and health spas. You do simple movements on the plate and the vibrating exercises the muscles. Jumping on small trampolines can be fun and give you a good workout too.

Your weight alone is not an indicator of good health because it does not distinguish between pounds that come from body fat and those that come from lean body mass or muscle. Muscle weighs more than fat. You can weigh almost the same as your trainer but she has more muscle and you probably have more fat. Muscles burn calories.

Carrying too much fat causes a condition called obesity and this condition puts a person at risk for many serious medical problems such as high blood pressure, diabetes, stroke, and heart disease. Overweight means an excess of total body weight based on population averages for height and body frame sizes.

Women have more body fat that men - about 10% more. By nature, a woman's body is developed to protect her and a potential fetus. As a result, women have more enzymes for storing fat and fewer enzymes for burning fat. Additionally, the estrogen women have activates fat storing enzymes and causes them to multiply. A drop in estrogen can cause a fat cell to become seven times larger because it is trying to make more estrogen. Women experience more changes in hydration levels than men because of their menstrual cycle. Changes in hydration levels can also be due to food, caffeine or alcohol consumption, strenuous exercise, stress or illness, or the taking of prescription drugs. Take weight and body fat measurements over a period of time to check progress.

Locate, borrow, or buy a BMI scale and measure your body composition; mass index, body fat, body water, muscle mass, bone mass, visceral fat, and metabolic age with it. On the Internet you can find various charts showing the BMI's for men and women of different ages and the health risks for the different categories.

Posture:

Very few people are aware of their posture when they are standing and walking. So many aches and pains in your body are caused by poor posture. A back pain may actually come from lack of arch support in your shoes, walking toes in or like a duck, unstable knees or hips. Walking with one shoulder higher than the other, standing twisted, sitting badly supported, tailbone alignment being off can cause problems. Chiropractors or physicians can help you identify where the problems might be coming from.

Cardio:

Your heart is also a muscle and need just as much exercise as every other muscle in your body. Raising your heart rate for 15 minutes a day is very beneficial.

Weight training: Working out with small bar bells or larger ones can help all ages build muscles and retain bone mass. It is better to increase repetitions not increase weight as much. Muscles get damaged when you work with too much weight.

Cross training: Doing the same type of exercises over and over doesn't exercise as many muscles as cross training. Mix your routine up a little. Swim, bike, walk the dog, paddle a kayak or canoe, play a racquet game, dance around the house, walk up and down the stairs.

SOURCES

Chapter #1- You Are What You Eat
<u>The Food Revolution</u> by John Robbins

<u>The China Study</u> by T. Collin Campbell, PhD & Thomas M. Campbell II
<u>Forks Over Knives</u> by T. Collin Campbell, PhD & Caldwell B. Esselstyn, Jr., MD
<u>Healthy Eating, Healthy World</u> by Jim Hicks

T. Collin Campbell, PhD was educated at Penn State, Cornell and MIT. He has consulted as a senior science advisor to the American Institute for Cancer Research, has been a member of several National Academy of Sciences expert panels on food and health, and currently sits on the advisory board of the Physicians Committee for Responsible Medicine. He is a professor Emeritus of Nutrition Biochemistry at Cornell University and the author of over 300 research papers.

Caldwell B. Esselstyn Jr., MD has been associated with the Cleveland Clinic since 1968 and has served as the chair of its breast cancer task force, chair of its thyroid and parathyroid surgery department. Today, he runs the cardiovascular prevention and reversal program at the clinic's Wellness Institute. He has written more than 150 scientific articles and wrote Prevent and Reverse Heart Disease as well as co-authored **Forks over Knives** with T. Collin Campbell.

Neal Barnard, MD is an adjunct professor of medicine at the George Washington University in Washington D.C. and a researcher funded by the National Institutes of Health. He is also the author of more than 15 books on nutrition and health as well as journal articles. He is the president of the Physicians Committee for Responsible Medicine.

John A. McDougall, MD has been studying and writing books on the effects of nutrition on disease for more than thirty years. He has dedicated his life to urging the public to eat a high starch, plant based diet. He is the founder and medical director of the McDougall Program, a residential treatment center in Santa Rosa, CA.

Dr. Joseph Mercola went to the University of Illinois and is a licensed physician and surgeon specializing in osteopathic medicine (which means treating the "whole person"). He is on the advisory board of the American Nutrition association, has written numerous articles and several health related books, and appears on TV as a guest expert in nutrition.

John Robbins is the son of Baskin-Robbins ice cream founder Irving Robbins. He grew up on a dairy and ate a lot of ice cream in his youth "for the company". He did his undergraduate studies at Berkeley and his masters at Antioch College. His first book, <u>Diet for a New America</u> (1987), advocated a "plant based, vegan diet and was nominated for the Pulitzer Prize. It contained his views on the meat and dairy industries, world hunger and human health. In the book, <u>Food Revolution</u>, that followed in 2001, he updated his ideas. John has received the Rachel Carson Award and the Albert Schweitzer Humanitarian Award among other awards.

Center for Food Safety- True Food Shoppers' Guide to Avoiding GMO's This app is available for iPhone and Android or download it to your computer.

<u>Salt Your Way to Health</u> by Dr. David Brownstein

What fish to eat: Monterey Bay Aquarium Seafood Watch pocket guides which can be downloaded on to your computer and there is also an app for the i phone or Android

Mediterranean diet pyramid of foods is available on the Internet.

<u>The Grain Brain</u> by David Perlmutter, MD

<u>Wheat Belly</u> by William Davis

<u>From Sugar to Splenda</u> by Professor Bert Fraser Reid

Dr. Lita Lee, PhD <u>Health Effects of Microwave Radiation- Microwave Ovens</u>

Chapter #2 Your Health

Dr. Lita Lee, PhD is a chemist, enzyme therapist, nutritionist, author and lecturer and has been in private practice since 1984.

Dr. Ray Peat, PhD has a PhD in biology from the University of Oregon with a specialization in physiology. He has taught at the following schools: University of Oregon, Urbana College, Montana State University, National College of Naturopathic Medicine, Universidad Veracruzana, Universidad Autonoma del Estado de Mexico and Blake College. He started his work with progesterone and related hormones in 1968. Over the years in various papers, he outlined his ideas regarding progesterone, and the hormones closely related to it as protectors of the body's structure and energy against the harmful effect of estrogen, radiation, stress, and lack of oxygen. The key idea was that energy and structure are interdependent at every level.

Dr. John R. Lee, MD was internationally acknowledged as a pioneer and expert in the study and use of the hormone progesterone, and on the subject of hormone replacement therapy for women. He graduated from Harvard and the University of Minnesota Medical School. After retiring from a thiry year family practice in Northern California, he began writing and traveling around the world speaking to doctors, scientists and lay people about progesterone. He wrote several books on women's health before his death in 2003.

Anticancer- A New Way of Life by David Servan-Schreiber, MD, PhD
Dr. Servan-Schreiber was co founder and then director of the Centre for Integrative Medicine at the University of Pittsburgh Medical Center. He was one of the founders of the U.S. branch of doctors without borders. At the age of 31, he was diagnosed with a malignant brain tumor and treated with the normal treatment of the day. He became a leading figure for integrative approaches to the prevention and treatment of cancer. He died in 2011 after almost 20 yrs of fighting a cancer considered to be terminal at the time of his diagnosis.

Prescription for Disaster DVD by Dr. Gary Null, PhD **Dr. Null** is an award winning American talk radio host and author who advocates for alternative medicine and naturopathy.

Marcelle Pick OB/GYN, NP, RNC- founder of the Women to Women Clinic in Maine is considered the premier for integrative care for women for over 25 years.

Dr. Russell Blaylock- a nationally recognized, board certified neurosurgeon, health practitioner, author, and lecturer.

Dr Daniel G. Amen- an American psychiatrist, a brain disorder specialist, director of the Amen Clinics, and a ten time New York Times best selling Author

<u>Sweet Remedy- The World Reacts to an Adulterated Food Supply</u>
This DVD is available from Amazon.

ADHD herbal remedies: www.NativeRemedies.com

The Great Cholesterol Myth by Dr. Jonny Bowden, Ph.D., C.N.S. and
Dr. Stephen Sinatra, M.D. F.A.C.C.

There is an exciting brand new book out now in 2017 by Dr. Dale Bredesen
on Alzheimer's called <u>The End of Alzheimer's</u>

Chapter #3- More Than Just Pampering
<u>The Touch of Healing</u> by Alice Burmeister

Reflexology: taking a new look" article by Christopher Shirley (owner/di-
rector of the Pacific Institute of Reflexology)

Reflexology- you can't beat the feet forum www.mothernature.com/
Library/Bookshelf/Books/21/42.cfm

Chapter #4- Our Toxic Environment
Nuclear information and resource service www.nirs.org

DoSomething.org

Humane Society of the United States 2015

Natural Resources Defense Council 2015

<u>Toxic Nation</u> by Fred Setterberg & Dr. Lonny Shavelson

The Breast Cancer-Pesticide Connection by Dr. Lita Lee

Detoxify or Die by Sherry A. Rogers, MD

Sheri Rogers, MD is a leading, nationally recognized, toxicologist who has written many books on various toxin related subjects. She has been in private practice for over 26 years.

Staying Well in a Toxic World by Lynn Lawson

Lynn Lawson grew up in rural Wisconsin and went to college where she received a BS in chemistry. Forty years later, she discovered that her increasingly severe headaches were caused by her diet and environment. Once she learned what chemicals and foods to avoid, how to avoid them, and how to build up her immune system, her health improved dramatically.

Nontoxic and Natural by Debra Lynn Dadd

Debra Lynn Dadd called the "Queen of Green" by the NY Times and is the author of six environmental consumer guidebooks.

Chapter #5- Detoxing
Environmental Working Group (EWG)- shopper's guide to the Dirty Dozen and the Clean Fifteen fruits and vegetables

Chapter #6- Use It or Loose It
Tanita.com- scales to measure Body Mass Index and more

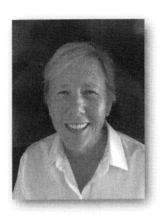

When she was a teenager, Wendy Richards used to tease her mother about attending "witch doctor" classes—courses on alternative medicine. But watching her mother live into her nineties with remarkably good health made Richards a firm believer in alternative therapies.

By changing her diet, lifestyle and opting for medical doctors who also used alternative medical knowledge in their practices, Richards improved her health dramatically: her allergies vanished, her gum problems improved, and colds became a rare occurrence, etc. She was able to take a more prevention position with her own health. In *Your Health in America*, which she has spent the past ten years compiling and streamlining, Richards passes on to you this vital alternative knowledge in hopes of initiating a positive trend in your health and quality of life.

INDEX

Made in the USA
Columbia, SC
17 January 2018